Surgical Atlas of Functional Single Ventricle and Hypoplastic Left Heart Syndrome

Bin Qiao • Zhong Min Liu
Yu Guo Weng • Ajit P. Yoganathan
Editors

Surgical Atlas of Functional Single Ventricle and Hypoplastic Left Heart Syndrome

PEOPLE'S MEDICAL PUBLISHING HOUSE

Springer

Editors
Bin Qiao
Cardiovascular Institute
General Hospital of Jinan Military Region
Jinan
China

Cardiac Surgery Center
Western District of Shandong
Provincial Hospital
Jinan
China

Yu Guo Weng
German Heart Center Berlin
Berlin
Germany

Zhong Min Liu
Shanghai Dongfang Hospital
Tongji University
Shanghai
China

Ajit P. Yoganathan
Wallace H. Coulter Department of
Biomedical Engineering
Georgia Institute of Technology
and Emory University
Atlanta
Georgia
USA

Jointly published with People's Medical Publishing House

ISBN 978-981-13-4150-2 ISBN 978-981-10-8435-5 (eBook)
https://doi.org/10.1007/978-981-10-8435-5

The print edition is not for sale in China Mainland. Customers from China Mainland please order the print book from: People's Medical Publishing House.

Printed on acid-free paper

This Springer imprint is published by the registered company Springer Nature Singapore Pte Ltd. part of Springer Nature
The registered company address is: 152 Beach Road, #21-01/04 Gateway East, Singapore 189721, Singapore

This book is dedicated to children with congenital heart disease and their families

and

All personnel engaged in the work of fighting congenital heart disease

Preface

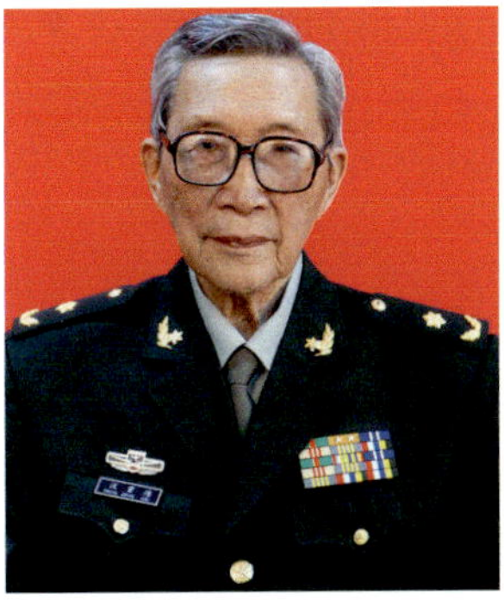

In recent years, many cardiac surgical atlases have come into being in China; however, there is still no atlas on complex congenital heart disease. It is rather difficult to operate on functional single ventricle and left ventricular hypoplasia syndromes, the former being widely addressed in China, while the latter is less common. Despite this difficulty, there is still a lack of a systematic and complete surgical atlas related to these syndromes. The chief editors, Bin Qiao, Zhong Min Liu, Yu Guo Weng, and Ajit P. Yoganathan, are specialists in the fields of cardiac surgery and biomedical engineering. They have compiled the book *Surgical Atlas of Functional Single Ventricle and Hypoplastic Left Heart Syndrome* by combining their clinical practical experience with the latest international developments.

As the old Chinese sayings go "A picture is worth a thousand words" and "Seeing is believing." This atlas, with a total of 202 color pictures and 56,000 words, brings together the wisdom and experience of the editors; it is based on clinical cardiac needs and more clearly reflects both anatomical morphology and surgical procedures and precautions due to its combination with current clinical practice. This atlas is illustrated concisely and clearly to be convenient for a majority of clinicians, cardiac surgeons, and medical teachers and students.

Furthermore, the addition of the fluid mechanics section is intended to introduce the cutting-edge concepts and techniques related to the optimization of the surgical process. I believe that the realization of operative simulations and assessments will rapidly develop the field of heart surgery.

The atlas includes novel topics and exciting content that have been condensed by the editors who have many years of valuable clinical experience. I am convinced that the publication of this atlas will be welcomed by readers, so I am writing this preface to recommend the book!

Jinan, China
Nov, 2014

Zengwei Wang

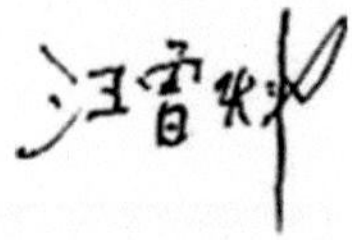

Contents

About the Editors

Bin Qiao, M.D.

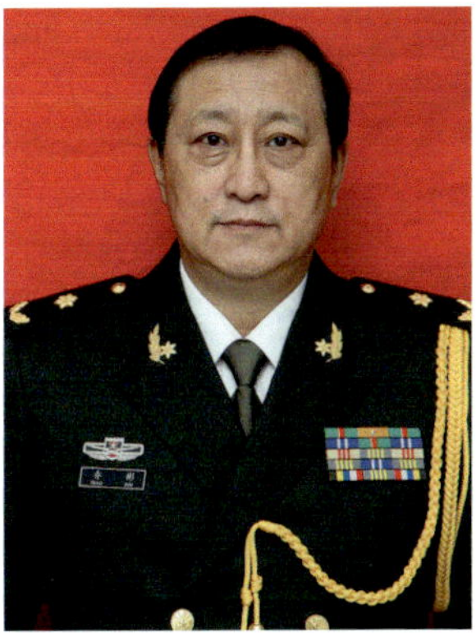

is the chief surgeon, professor, and doctoral supervisor in the Cardiovascular Institute of Jinan Military District. He is also the director of the Chinese PLA Pediatric Cardiovascular Center and a senior advisor to the *Chinese Journal of Thoracic and Cardiovascular Surgery* and *Chinese Journal of Extracorporeal Circulation*. He has dedicated over three decades to the field of complex congenital heart disease repair and has made numerous innovatory achievements in the field.

In 2001, Dr. Qiao successfully performed interventional therapy for a pediatric atrial septal defect assisted by 3D ultrasonic imaging. In 2005, he performed the first successful infant allograft heart transplantation in China. In 2009, he proposed the bilateral bidirectional Glenn and incomplete Fontan operations and utilized them to treat single ventricle patients unsuitable for the conventional Fontan operation. In 2011, to prevent trauma from sternal incisions, he proposed the use of minimally invasive surgery for complex congenital heart diseases, and this method was successfully applied as a surgical treatment for more than twenty subcategories of complex congenital heart diseases, including the Tetralogy of Fallot, double outlet right ventricle, and double chambered right ventricle. Starting in 2014, he employed cardiovascular simulation to plan and design surgeries. With this technique, he strives to renovate the extracardiac Fontan procedure and make groundbreaking progress in the physiological correction of functional single ventricles.

Zhong Min Liu, Ph.D., M.D.

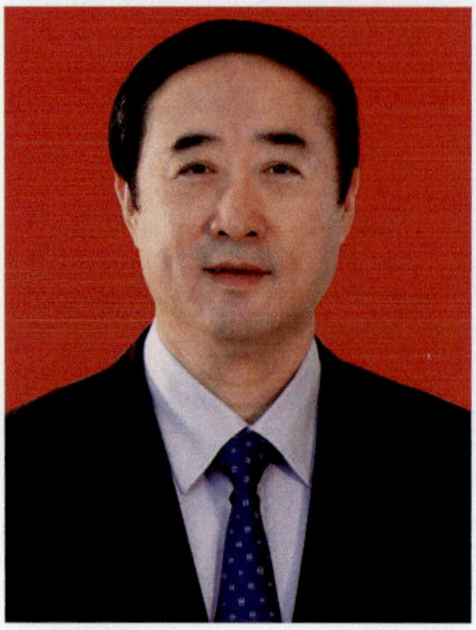

is the chief surgeon, professor, and doctoral advisor in the Shanghai East Hospital. Additionally, he is the president of the Shanghai Dongfang Hospital, an expert enjoying special government allowances of the State Council, a joint professor of the fifth University of Paris, France, and a vice president of the cardiovascular surgery branch of the Chinese medical doctor association.

Dr. Liu has been devoted to the research and clinical practice of thoracic and cardiovascular surgery for more than 35 years and specializes in a variety of complex, difficult congenital heart diseases, including rheumatic valvular disease, coronary heart disease, vascular disease, lung cancer, and esophageal cancer. He is one of the pioneers in the use of artificial heart devices and the performance of heart and lung transplantations to treat heart failure in China. He leads more than ten projects which are funded by national level funds, such as the 863 program of the national Natural Science Foundation of China. He holds the position as the deputy director of the cardiovascular surgery division of the Chinese Medical Doctor Association.

Dr. Liu has studied in Japan, the United States, Germany, Denmark, and many other countries and obtained a European medical license issued by the German Heart Center with his rigorous style and skilled surgical technique.

Dr. Liu has published more than 150 papers, including thirty-three SCI papers. He is editor-in-chief for eight published books. He has been awarded the second prize of the Chinese Medical Science and Technology Award, as well as many other honors. He owns more than six practical invention patents.

Yu Guo Weng, M.D.

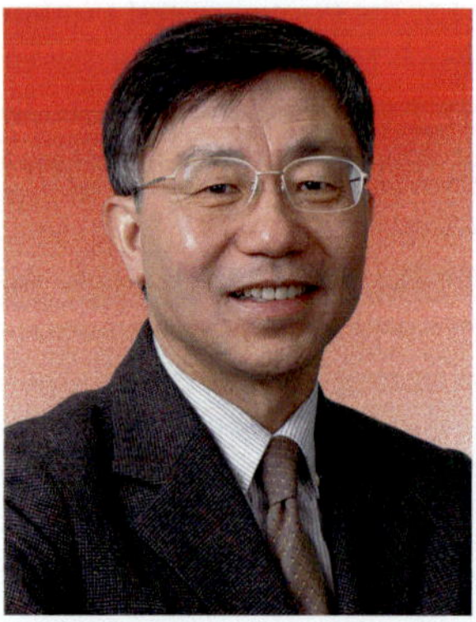

is the vice chairman and the chief physician of the German Heart Center Berlin and has been a professor at Humboldt University since 1987. He is a member of the German Association of Cardiothoracic Surgery. He was the editor and reviewer of the *Asian Journal of Cardiothoracic Surgery*, the *American Journal of Thoracic Surgery*, and the *Chinese Journal of Cardiovascular Research*. He is an honorary professor at the Second Military Medical University, the Third Military Medical University, and the Fourth Military Medical University. He was a visiting professor at Shanghai Second Medical University, East Hospital (affiliated with Tongji University), Peking Hospital (affiliated with Peking University), Guangdong Cardiovascular Institute, Fujian Medical University, Jiangsu University of Science and Technology, Zhenjiang Medical College, Medical School of Ningbo University, Zhongshan Medical University, Lanzhou Medical College, Qingdao Medical College, and Jinan University. He is the surgical consultant of Shenyang Military Region General Hospital.

Being a senior cardiac surgeon, he has performed surgical operations for more than 10,000 cases involving a variety of complex congenital heart diseases, including large blood vessels, heart valves, coronary heart disease, heart transplantations, heart and lung transplantations, and cardiac assist devices. He was awarded the Special Contribution by the Chinese Medical Association of Cardiothoracic Surgery in 2010. His achievements are selectively summarized here: switch operations in neonates since 1984, homologous aortic grafts since 1986, heart and heart-lung transplantations since 1987, ventricular assist devices since 1989, latissimus dorsi dynamic cardiomyopathy in 1990, four-valve replacement in one patient in 1993, end-stage dilated cardiomyopathy cured by ventricular assist device in 1994, TAPVC radical surgery for a 1.6 kg premature infant in 1995, robotic surgery since 1999, total artificial hearts since 1999, and end-stage heart failure treated with stem cells since 2004, as well as many others.

Ajit P. Yoganathan

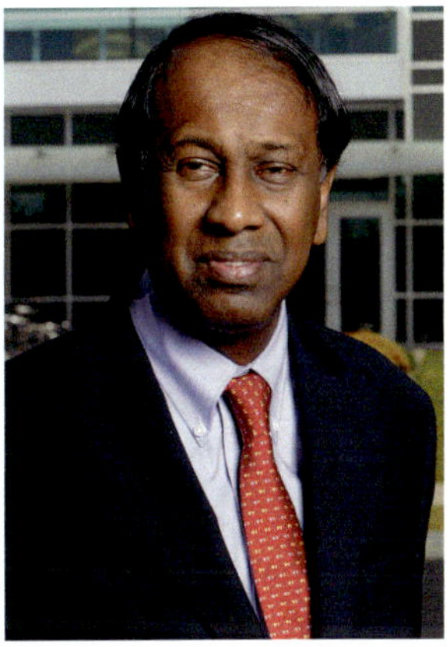

For more than 40 years. Ajit P. Yoganathan has been a pioneer in basic and translational cardiovascular research, especially experimental and computational fluid mechanics as it pertains to artificial heart valves, the whole heart, and congenital heart diseases. His work involves the use of optical techniques such as laser Doppler velocimetry, digital particle image velocimetry, computational fluid dynamics, and clinical tools such as cardiac ultrasound and magnetic resonance imaging to noninvasively study and quantify blood flow patterns and parameters in the cardiovascular system, both on the bench, in silico, and in vivo. In an effort to take an interdisciplinary and translational approach to his research, Dr. Yoganathan has established collaborations with clinicians, scientists, and industry professionals worldwide.

Dr. Yoganathan received a Bachelor of Science and a Doctor of Philosophy in Chemical Engineering in 1973 from University College, University of London, and in 1978 from the California Institute of Technology, respectively. Since joining the Georgia Tech faculty in 1979, Dr. Yoganathan has mentored more than 50 doctoral students, 35 master's students, and 30 postdoctoral trainees. He played a pivotal role in the creation of Georgia Tech's master's and Ph.D. degree programs in bioengineering as well as the joint Ph.D. in biomedical engineering with the Emory University School of Medicine. In 2010, he was appointed the founding editor-in-chief of Cardiovascular Engineering and Technology (CVET)—one of the newest journals of the Biomedical Engineering Society which in 2015 was accepted to PubMed. His many distinguished honors include the Alexander von Humboldt Fellowship from West Germany (1985), the H.R. Lissner Award from the American Society of Mechanical Engineers (1997), the Pritzker Lecturer Award from the Biomedical Engineering Society (2012), the Ann Newman Lecturer Award from the Children's Hospital of Philadelphia (2012), and elected membership to the prestigious National Academy of Engineering in Washington, DC (2015). Since 2005 when he was appointed Chair of the Cardiovascular SubCommittee of the International Standards Organization Technical Committee on Implants for Surgery, Dr. Yoganathan has also played an important role in the development of US and international standards for cardiovascular devices. In recognition of this, the Association for the Advancement of Medical Instrumentation presented him with Standards Developer Award in 2015. He currently has 10 issued US patents—with more than a dozen applications—and to date has published more than 40 book chapters and 400 peer-reviewed journal articles (more than 50 regarding congenital single ventricle defects). It is worth noting that all prosthetic heart valves in use in the United States since 1975 have been evaluated—either directly or indirectly— in Dr. Yoganathan's Cardiovascular Fluid Mechanics Lab.

Introduction

Functional single ventricle is a cyanotic complex congenital heart disease with varied pathological types. For more than a decade, the Heart and Disease Society of Europe and the United States have proposed a categorical and surgical guideline for congenital heart disease, formalizing its naming system. Surgical treatment has also been standardized as a staged Fontan surgery, establishing a serial circulation by bypassing the right ventricle. However, the Fontan surgery is, after all, a palliative approach, and postoperative complications, Fontan circulation failure, and risk factors have not been fully understood or effectively treated. Left ventricular hypoplasia syndrome belongs to the pathological category of functional single ventricle disorders; its lesions are more complex and critical, and children with this disease often die shortly after birth. Final surgical treatment for left ventricular hypoplasia syndrome resorts to a modified Fontan surgery, and the Norwood procedure is divided into three stages. A definitive diagnosis, operative procedure, and perioperative management are difficult to determine, and various postoperative complications and Fontan function failure are likely to occur. The surgical treatment of left ventricular hypoplasia syndrome is limited to a handful of hospitals in the world and is almost nonexistent in China. The editors have been engaged in the treatment of the disease for several decades, have experienced much of the developmental process of operative techniques for single ventricle malformations, and have altogether accumulated hundreds of surgical cases. We are therefore responsible for the preparation of this atlas on functional single ventricle and left heart hypoplasia syndrome. It is difficult to elaborate in words the classification, pathophysiology, and surgical methods of the diseases, so this book is presented in the form of illustrations. All pictures have been illustrated by the surgeons themselves. Liping Zhu, professor in the Department of Anatomy at Shandong University, has refined the pictures.

This book is divided into three parts.

Part I introduces the basic concepts of functional single ventricles, the history of surgical treatment, the evolution of various surgeries, and the current standard staged modified Fontan surgery. The fundamental reason for Fontan circulation failure is the lack of power in the pulmonary circulation, and it is necessary for many experts to provide a long-term available power source for the Fontan circulation. The editors proposed two innovative ideas and surgical methods to improve power sources for modified Fontan circulation based on their own clinical experience and hope that the techniques will be shared with readers and improved in the future.

Part II specially introduces left ventricular hypoplasia syndrome; the contents and additional illustrations are arranged according to the German classification guidelines of congenital heart disease. Heart transplantation may be the best approach to an anatomical treatment of left ventricular hypoplasia syndrome.

Part III summarizes the applications and research progress of cardiovascular simulation in the field of cardiovascular surgery. The hemodynamic characteristics of Qiao's modified bidirectional Glenn shunt and Qiao's incomplete Fontan operation are given as examples in this section for clinical reference.

Fontan surgery has had 40 years of history, and there are a variety of methods that have improved the original procedure. This book provides a brief introduction to some typical, historic operations; some rare cases such as double outlet left or right ventricle, imbalanced atrioventricular septal defect, functional single ventricle with atrial heterogeneity, neonatal functional single ventricle with subaortic stenosis (systemic ventricular outflow tract obstruction), and their surgical methods such as Damus–Kaye–Stansel are not detailed in this book. The reconstruction of a systemic to pulmonary shunt for failed Fontan circulation is also omitted. With its rapid development, it is also possible to incorporate hybridization or interventional therapies into staged Fontan surgery or Norwood surgery to treat functional single ventricle and left ventricular hypoplasia syndromes; however, these therapies are also not outlined in this book.

Special thanks should be given to my mentor, Prof Zengwei Wang, a grandmaster of heart surgery, for his great support and attention to the compilation of this atlas. He has reviewed the contents and written the preface for this book.

Many thanks also go to Dr. Zhenglun Alan Wei in Georgia Institute of Technology, Dr. Biao Si, Professor Tongjian Wang, and Dr. Na Li from the General Hospital of Jinan Military Region, for the editing and revision of the text of this book.

Due to limited experience and time, there will undoubtedly be a lot of shortcomings and errors. We hope that readers can give their comments and suggestions to the editors so that the book can be improved in future editions.

Jinan, China
Shanghai, China
Berlin, Germany
Atlanta, GA, USA
November, 2017

Bin Qiao,
Zhong Min Liu,
Yu Guo Weng,
Ajit P. Yoganathan,

Part I
Functional Single Ventricle

Chapter 1
Etiologic Classification of Diseases

Bin Qiao and Hong Yan Wang

Single ventricle (SV) is a complex congenital heart disease characterized by the formation of only one single functional ventricle during fetal development. The various malformations will result in different pathological blood circulation routes in single ventricle disease, so treatment methods must also vary. The basic pathological deformities consist of: a single ventricle that receives blood from the two atria, possibly paired with an additional small ventricle that is underdeveloped and only receives blood from the main ventricle. In fact, the heart in patients with SV only has one ventricle large enough to sustain the functions of systemic and pulmonary circulation. Other criteria for the diagnosis of the single ventricle include the relationship between the inflow or outflow tracts of the ventricle and the location of the atrioventricular valve, the connection between the great arteries and the single ventricle, and the relationship between the locations of the great arteries, which can be normal or transposed. Therefore, there are only two kinds of basic pathological forms of SV: the left ventricle presides over the systemic circulation and incidentally assists in lung circulation; on the contrary, the right ventricle is dominated presiding over the pulmonary circulation and incidentally assisting systemic circulation. So International Nomenclature and Database System for Congenital Heart Surgery named the disease as functional single ventricle (Jacobs and Mayer 2000). In principle, a separation operation cannot be performed on a functional single ventricle by surgery. Following this original classification, different names of the functional single ventricle based on its etiological diagnosis in the clinic are listed below:

B. Qiao (✉)
Cardiovascular Institute, General Hospital of Jinan Military Region, Jinan, China

Cardiac Surgery Center, Western District of Shandong Provincial Hospital, Jinan, China

H. Y. Wang
Department of Life Science, Fudan University, Shanghai, China

B. Qiao et al. (eds.), *Surgical Atlas of Functional Single Ventricle and Hypoplastic Left Heart Syndrome*, https://doi.org/10.1007/978-981-10-8435-5_1

1. Double inlet left ventricle. Two atrioventricular valves or a common atrioventricular valve connects with the functional left ventricle.
2. Double inlet right ventricle. Two atrioventricular valves or a common atrioventricular valve connects with the functional right ventricle.
3. Double outlet left ventricle. A great artery originates solely from the functional left ventricle and the other great arteries carry over 50% of the functional left ventricle.
4. Double outlet right ventricle. Two great arteries primarily or completely originate from the right ventricle.
5. Tricuspid atresia.
6. Mitral atresia. It is classified into hypoplasia left heart syndrome.
7. Pulmonary atresia with an intact ventricular septum.
8. Left ventricle-based single ventricle (Hypoplastic right ventricle).
9. Right ventricle-based single ventricle (Hypoplastic left heart syndrome, HLHS).

Reference

Jacobs ML, Mayer JE. Congenital heart surgery nomenclature and database project: single ventricle. Ann Thorac Surg. 2000;69(3):197–204. https://doi.org/10.1016/S0003-4975(99)01245-X.

Chapter 2
Anatomical Features

Bin Qiao and Na Li

A double inlet left ventricle is the most common subtype of double inlet ventricles, in which the predominate ventricle is the left ventricular structure (Fig. 2.1). Anatomical features consist of:

1. Two atrioventricular valves or a common atrioventricular valve that is directly connected to the left ventricular main chamber
2. Transposition of great arteries (TGA)
3. Transposition of left and right ventricles
4. Small right ventricle with dysplasia
5. Ventricular septal defect
6. Atrial septal defect
7. The aortic arch is further to the left than normal

A double inlet right ventricle is the right ventricular type of double inlet ventricles, in which the predominate ventricle is the right ventricular structure (Fig. 2.2). Anatomical features consist of:

1. Two atrioventricular valves or a common atrioventricular valve that is directly connected to the right ventricular main chamber.
2. The left and right atria are connected with the morphologic right ventricle.
3. Undeveloped left ventricle is located in the upper posterior of the dominant right ventricular chamber.

B. Qiao (✉)
Cardiovascular Institute, General Hospital of Jinan Military Region, Jinan, China

Cardiac Surgery Center, Western District of Shandong Provincial Hospital, Jinan, China

N. Li
Institute of Cardiovascular Diseases, Jinan Military Region General Hospital of PLA, Jinan, China

B. Qiao et al. (eds.), *Surgical Atlas of Functional Single Ventricle and Hypoplastic Left Heart Syndrome*, https://doi.org/10.1007/978-981-10-8435-5_2

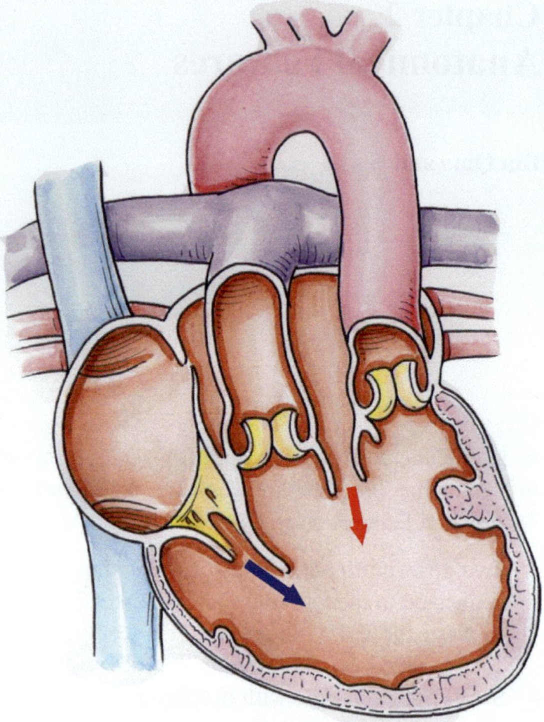

Fig. 2.1 Double inlet left ventricle

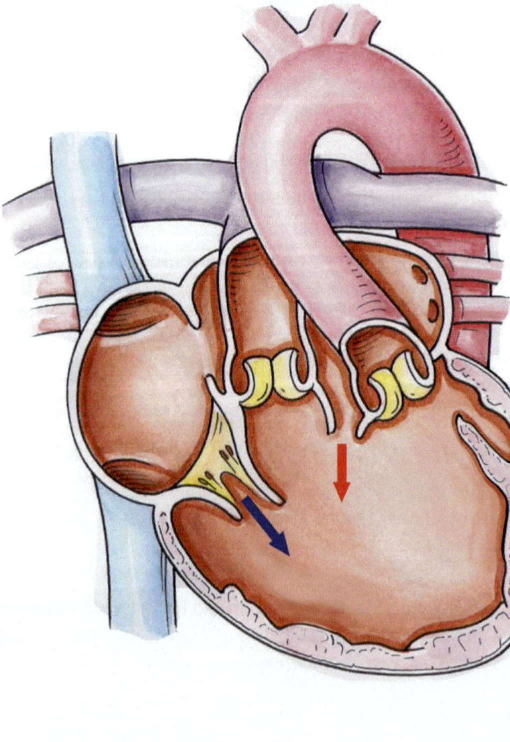

Fig. 2.2 Double inlet right ventricle

4. The undeveloped ventricle is often connected with the dominant ventricle through a very small ventricular septal defect.
5. Generally, there is no obvious great artery outflow tract.
6. The relationship of the great arteries is normal, or with left or right great arterial malposition; a double inlet right ventricle paired with an inconsistent connection between the ventricle and great arteries is rare.
7. It is common in double inlet right ventricles that the two arteries often originate from the main chamber of the right ventricle, or with pulmonary atresia.

By definition, tricuspid atresia (TA) includes tricuspid valve agenesis, no direct connection between the right atrium and the single ventricle, and right ventricle hypoplasia. Some pathologists place it in the same class as double inlet left ventricles with only the mitral valve between the left atrium and the left ventricle, accompanied by the hypertrophy of the left ventricle and mitral valves (Fig. 2.3). There are three types of pathological classification:

Type I is characterized by normal great artery relations, of which there are three subtypes:

(a) Pulmonary artery atresia
(b) Pulmonary artery hypoplasia associated with a small ventricular septal defect
(c) Normal pulmonary artery with a large ventricular septal defect

Type II is characterized by a right-sided aorta, of which there are also three subtypes:

(a) Pulmonary atresia
(b) Pulmonary arterial stenosis or subvalvular pulmonary stenosis
(c) Pulmonary artery expansion

Type IIIa is characterized by a left-sided aorta and includes two subtypes:

(a) Pulmonary arterial stenosis or subvalvular pulmonary stenosis
(b) Subaortic stenosis

Like tricuspid valve atresia, mitral atresia has no left atrioventricular connection and actually almost no functional left ventricle; if combined with aortic atresia or stenosis, mitral atresia should be pathologically classified as hypoplastic left heart syndrome, which will be discussed in this book in regard to its diagnosis and surgical treatment.

There is a large variety of pathological varieties of functional single ventricles, each of which containing a different conduction system. We will look at a hypoplastic right ventricle as an example to explain the anatomy of its conduction system.

A left ventricle-based single ventricle is a common type of functional single ventricle, in which the left ventricle is the main ventricular structure. The aorta is located in front of the left pulmonary artery but is not associated with subaortic stenosis (Fig. 2.4).

The conduction system arises from the anterior atrioventricular node, which is located in the junction between the right atrial appendage and atrial septum. The conduction bundle descends along the pulmonary artery annulus to the right edge of the bulboventricular foramen and is divided into left and right bundle branches at the

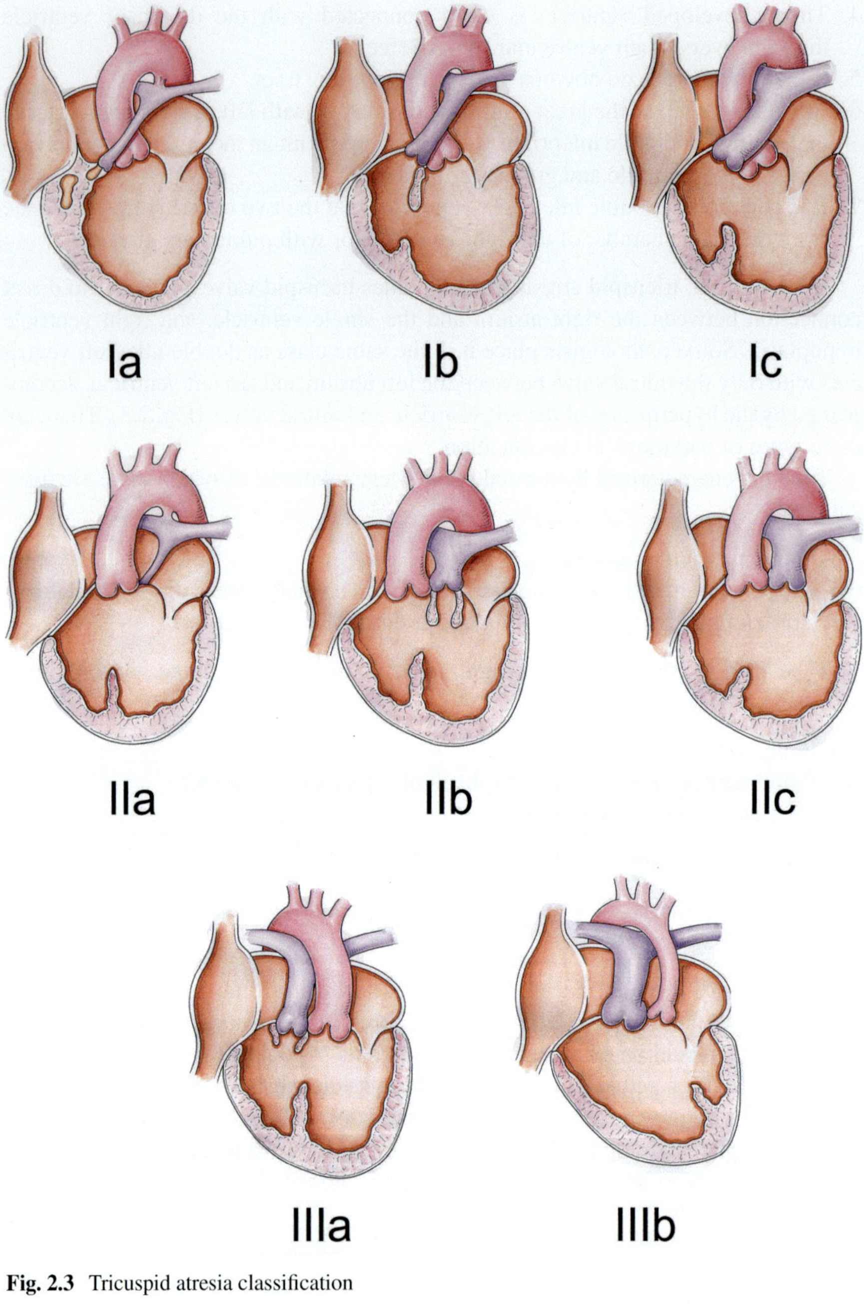

Fig. 2.3 Tricuspid atresia classification

muscle crest in the inferior edge of the bulboventricluar foramen. The left bundle branch advances into the primary ventricular chamber and right bundle branch into the crater cavity (Fig. 2.5).

A profound study performed by Anderson on the cardiac conduction bundle of single ventricles found that a single ventricle heart of van Praagh's type A has an

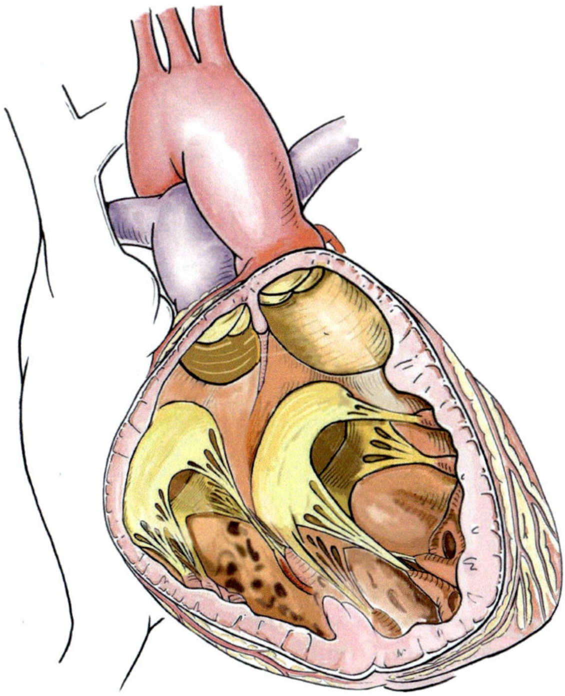

Fig. 2.4 Left ventricle-based single ventricle

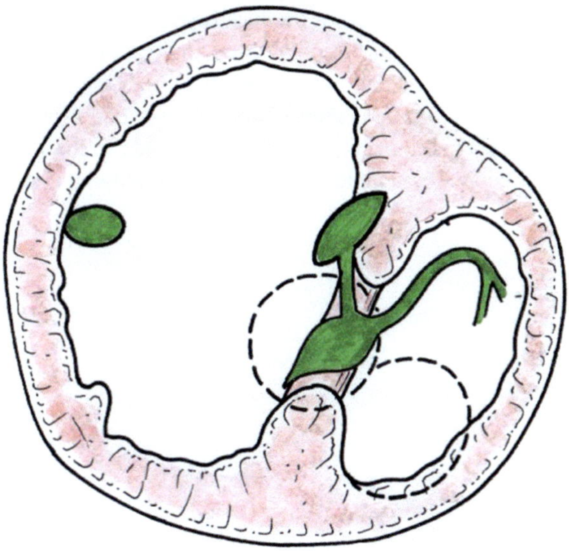

Fig. 2.5 Conduction system of functional single ventricle 1

undeveloped atrioventricular node at the posterior part of the atrial septum called a posterior node and another atrioventricular node called an anterior node in the connection between the right atrial appendage and the anterior atrial septum. The atrioventricular bundle arises from the anterior node. Along the outflow tract of the

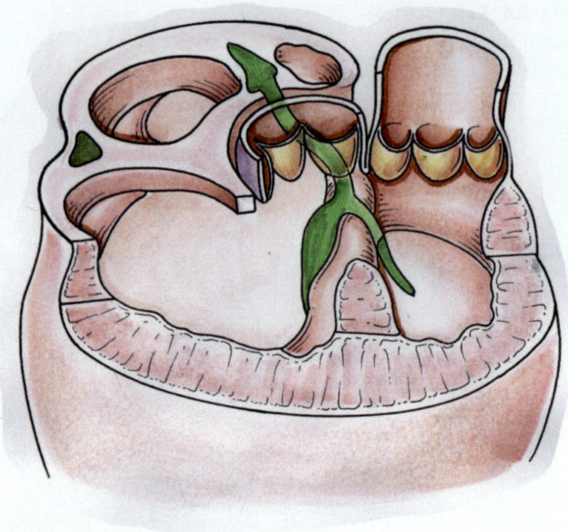

Fig. 2.6 Conduction system of functional single ventricle 2

rear large artery, which is the aortic valve if no transposition occurs, or else is the pulmonary valve, the atrioventricular bundle advances inferiorly to the right edge of the conical ventricle orifice and then is divided into a left and right bundle branch in the cone chamber ridge—the left bundle branch advances into the main cavity, while the right bundle branch goes to the residual cavity. This situation is the same for single ventricles of type IIa and type IIIa of van Praagh classification.

A sinus rhythm nerve impulse is sent from the anterior atrioventricular node and conducts along the conduction bundle from the infra-anterior to the posterior semilunar valve annulus to reach the upper edge of the conical chamber crest. The conduction bundle is then divided into left and right bundle branches at the top of the crest. The left bundle branch descends to the primary ventricular cavity while right bundle branch descends to the infundibular chamber (Fig. 2.6).

Chapter 3
Septation of the Single Ventricle: Corrective Surgery

Bin Qiao, Jing Huang, and Na Li

According to the International Congenital Heart Surgery Naming and Database System, a functional single ventricle in principle cannot be corrected by surgical septation operation. However, when historically used as a method to cure the single ventricle, successful cases show that in some appropriate patients with functional single ventricles, ventricular septation operations may be desirable. They are, after all, in the scope of radical surgery.

In 1956, Mayo clinic performed the first septation surgery on a single ventricle patient who was diagnosed with large artery transposition and with large ventricular septal defects. Single ventricle with transposed great arteries was found during operation. Therefore, a patch was placed in the single ventricle to separate it to two parts: one for systemic circulation, and the other one for pulmonary one. Although the survival time of the patient was not long, the septation surgery for single ventricle was deemed feasible. Due to difficulties in surgery, such as the choice of septal location in the main ventricle, the acquisition of a large enough patch, and the uncertainty of the postoperative survival rate, the use of the single ventricular septation surgery declined for more than ten years. In fact, the Mayo clinic did not perform a single ventricular septation surgery again until the 1970s. After that time, only a few number of cases had been reported over the next several decades. In general, patients often have a high mortality rate, postoperative residual ventricular septal defects, conduction blocks requiring pacemakers, and other common complications. Additionally, if patients had main pulmonary valve stenosis, reoperation had to be undertaken due to postoperative atrioventricular valve insufficiencies. The fact that

B. Qiao (✉)
Cardiovascular Institute, General Hospital of Jinan Military Region, Jinan, China

Cardiac Surgery Center, Western District of Shandong Provincial Hospital, Jinan, China

J. Huang · N. Li
Institute of Cardiovascular Diseases, Jinan Military Region General Hospital of PLA, Jinan, China

B. Qiao et al. (eds.), *Surgical Atlas of Functional Single Ventricle and Hypoplastic Left Heart Syndrome*, https://doi.org/10.1007/978-981-10-8435-5_3

only a small number of patients had satisfactory long-term outcomes daunted most heart surgeons. However, Dr. Ebert carried out the septation surgery in two stages in 1984 (Ebert 1984). In the first stage, the ventricular septal defect patch was divided into two parts, one of which was placed at the apical part, while the other was placed at the site between the semilunar valve and the atrioventricular valve; at the same time, the pulmonary artery was banded. In second stage, taking 6–18 months after first operation, the vacancy between the two previous ventricular septal defect patches was closed with a patch. Dr. Ebert reported few cases; although the results were satisfying, the new technology had not been widely popularized. In the 1980s, with the development of the cavopulmonary connection and the application of subsequent Fontan operations to create total cavopulmonary connections (TCPC), a common method currently for single ventricle surgeries, the use of septation surgeries faded away.

Prior to uniformly naming and classifying congenital heart disease, its various pathology types were often very vague. To ameliorate this issue, Van Praagh's method of single ventricle pathologic classification provides a valuable reference for its surgical treatment (Van Praagh 1992). According to the development of the single ventricle, it can be classified as type A, B, C, or D. Type A is classified as right ventricle sinus agenesis, in which only a residual cavity of the right ventricular infundibulum is connected to the single left ventricle. Type B is a left ventricular sinus agenesis, with only a single right ventricle. Type C is associated with undeveloped muscular ventricular septal defects and the development of both the left and right ventricular cavities. This type can also be understood as a complete ventricular septal defect or a common ventricle. In type D, the left and right ventricular sinuses and ventricular septum are all undeveloped. Furthermore, each type can be divided into I, II, III, and IV subtypes based on the corresponding relationships between the great arteries. Patients with subtype I have a normal relationship between the great arteries. In subtype II, the aorta is located in front of the right pulmonary artery and is called the right sided aorta. In subtype III, the aorta is located in front of the left pulmonary artery and is called the left sided aorta. Subtype IV is the mirror image of a normal great artery relationship. Thus, sixteen total basic types of single ventricle defects can be presented. This classification does not include relationships between the left and right atria, nor left pulmonary artery (LPA) stenosis, all of which should be additionally described in practice. Since the 1970s, a variety of single ventricle defects that belong to Type A III of Van Praagh's classification have been successfully corrected by a septation operation (Fig. 3.1). That is, the right ventricular sinus was undeveloped, one residual cavity of the right ventricular infundibulum was connected to the left single ventricle, and the aortic valve opening was located to the left and in front of the pulmonary valve opening.

The ideal indication of the single ventricle septation surgery is that in which the case has an undeveloped right ventricle with only a residual cavity connected to the left single ventricular chamber and that has a left translocated aorta in front of the left pulmonary artery, which causes the left ventricular outflow tract directly below it. These patients have intact mitral and tricuspid valves both in structure and function, without main pulmonary artery (MPA) stenosis. One common atrioventricular valve, very small ventricular cavity, or other severe malformations, such as interruption of the aortic arch, are contraindications of the septation surgery. The parallel blood flow direction of the pulmonary and systemic arteries ensures that the single ventricle can be repaired by septation surgery (Fig. 3.2).

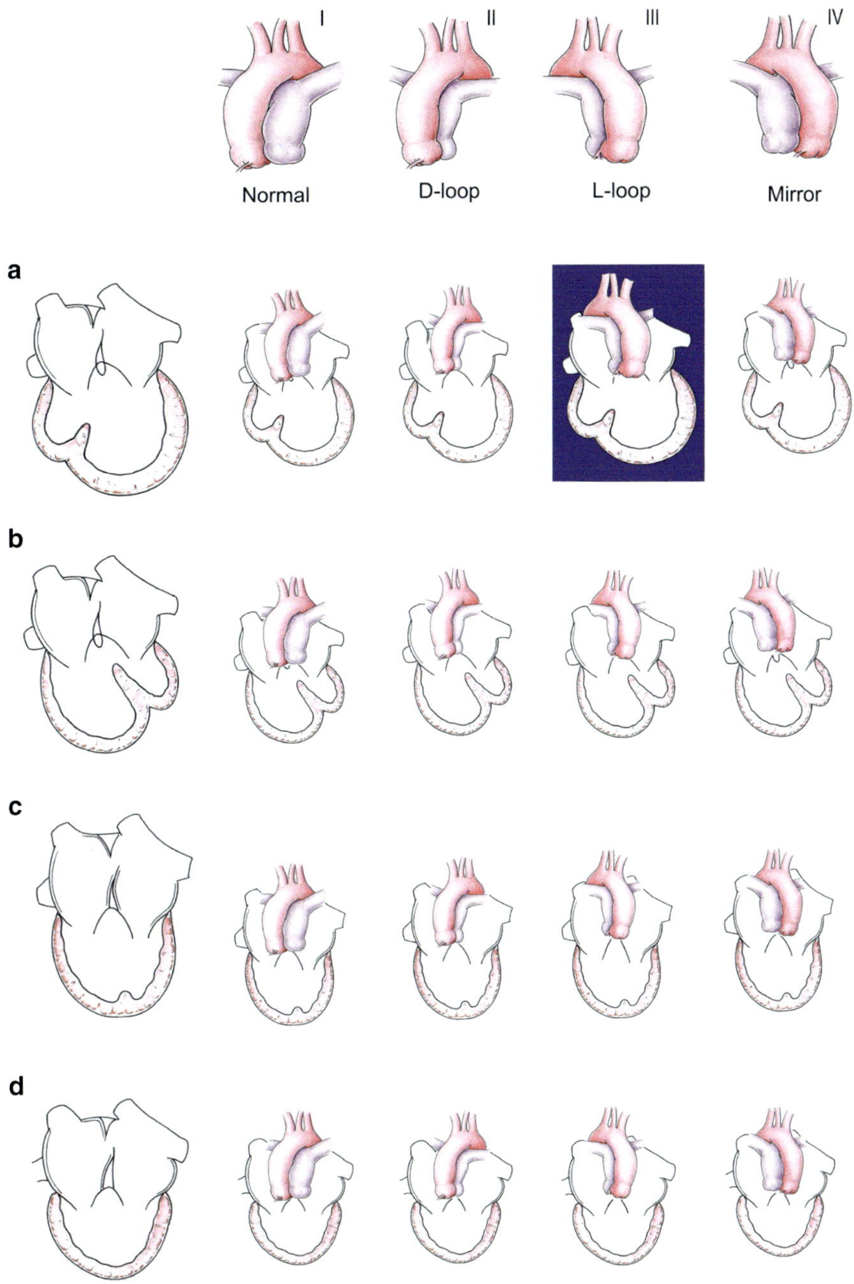

Fig. 3.1 Van Praagh classification of single ventricle

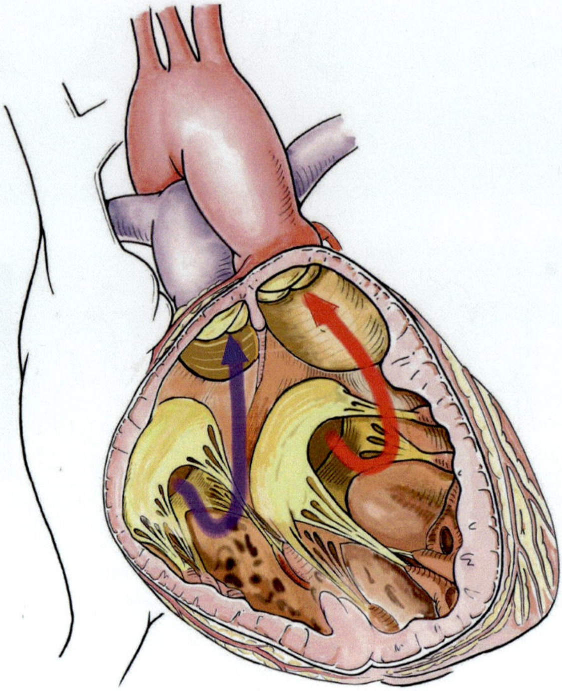

Fig. 3.2 Flow direction of AIII single ventricle

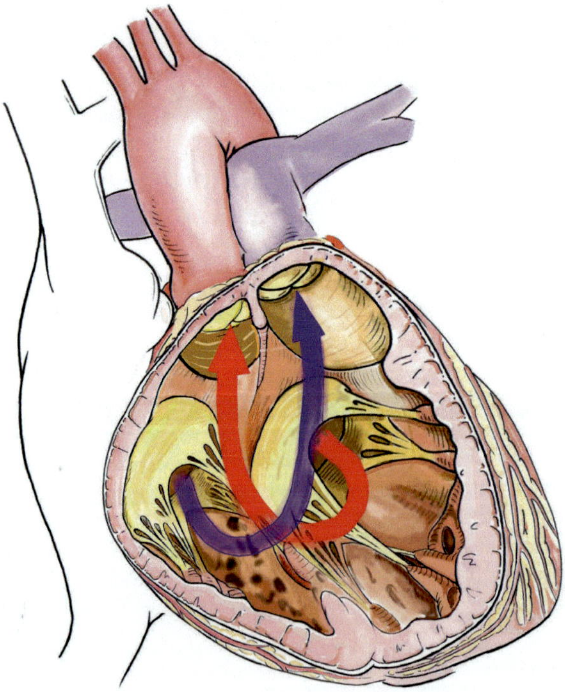

Fig. 3.3 Flow direction of AII type single ventricle

If the position of the pulmonary artery and aorta is transposed, the blood flow direction of the pulmonary and systemic arteries must cross each other. In these cases, a septation procedure cannot be performed (Fig. 3.3).

Most functional single ventricle cases are excluded by strict patient selection before septation surgery. Extracorporeal circulation is adopted in surgery under moderate hypothermia. Aortic cannulation is performed. The superior and inferior venae cavae (SVC and IVC) are directly intubated to drain venous blood. Cardiac preservation solution is routinely infused after blocking the ascending aorta. The difficulty of the septation operation lies in finding an appropriate septation point for the repair of the ventricular septal defect in the apical part of the single ventricle. Ventricular and atrial incisions are both made, which provides convenience in exposing and repairing the heart. Branches of the coronary arteries should be protected carefully. The dashed lines show the locations of the incisions (Fig. 3.4).

The Dacron patch, soft yet sturdy, is appropriate as a septal patch. The texture of expanded polytetrafluoroethylene (Gore-Tex) is hard and difficult to suture when tightened. Following the location of the apex of the ventricle and the determination of the septation point of the ventricular septum, repair was performed by interrupted polyene sutures with a small pad (Fig. 3.5).

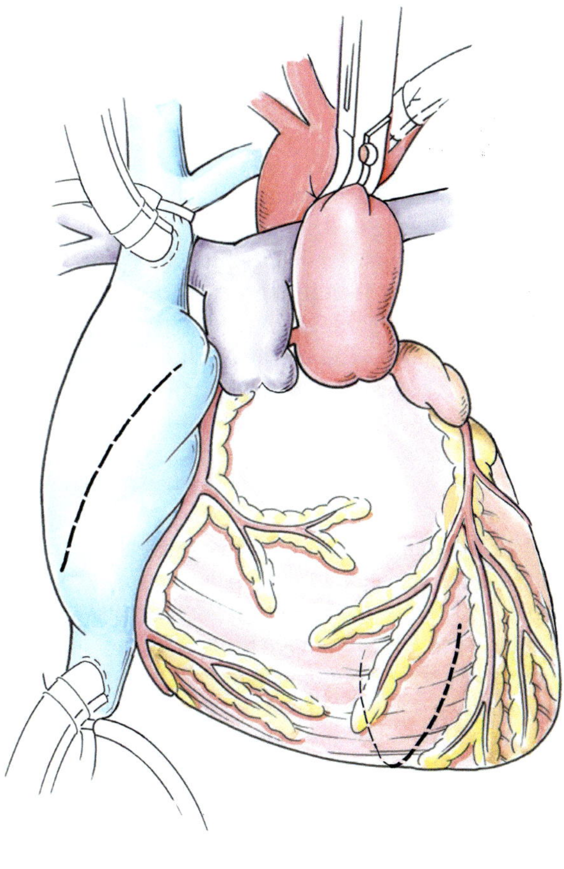

Fig. 3.4 Single ventricular septation surgery: incision

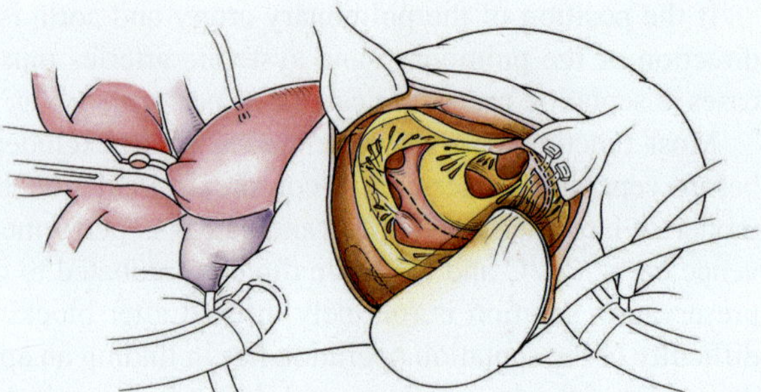

Fig. 3.5 Single ventricular septal surgery: patch position

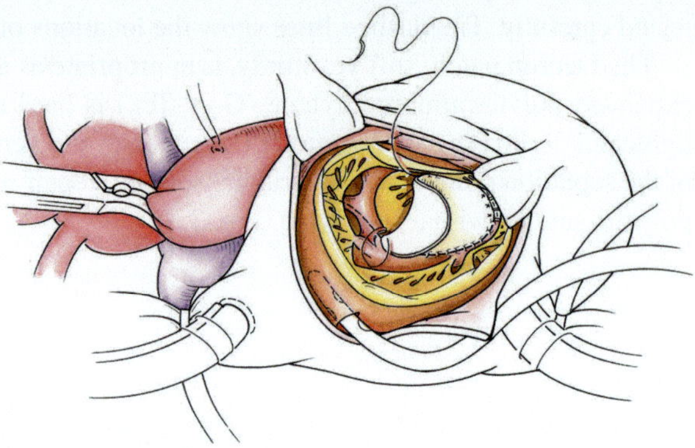

Fig. 3.6 Single ventricular septation surgery: the separation method

It is difficult yet important to identify the ventricular septum in a septation operation. The right atrial incision should be large enough to expose the entire ventricular cavity. After determining that the systemic and pulmonary artery blood flow is parallel by identifying the relationship between the main pulmonary valve and atrioventricular valve, the location between them can act as a septation location with a patch. The apical patch can be sewed with interrupted sutures and small pads, while the ventricular anterior and posterior walls should be sewed with a continuous method. During the separating procedure, the left ventricular cavity is maintained large enough to sustain the systemic circulation. The right ventricular cavity can be relatively smaller because it only sustains the pulmonary circulation (Fig. 3.6).

The relationships between the two great arterial valves and two atrioventricular valves make septation of the single ventricle feasible. The blood pathway through which oxygenated blood in the left atrium flows into the aorta through the atrioventricular valve orifice is called the arterial blood flow line, while the blood from the right atrium flowing into the pulmonary artery through the tricuspid valve is called the venous blood flow line. The arterial and venous blood flow lines are parallel to each other when the aortic and pulmonary valve orifices are directly next to each other, so just a piece of a tablet-like artificial patch can completely separate the two blood flows in surgery. However, if the flows intersect in the heart, septation surgery cannot be performed. In a scenario that no trabecular muscle or muscle ridge is

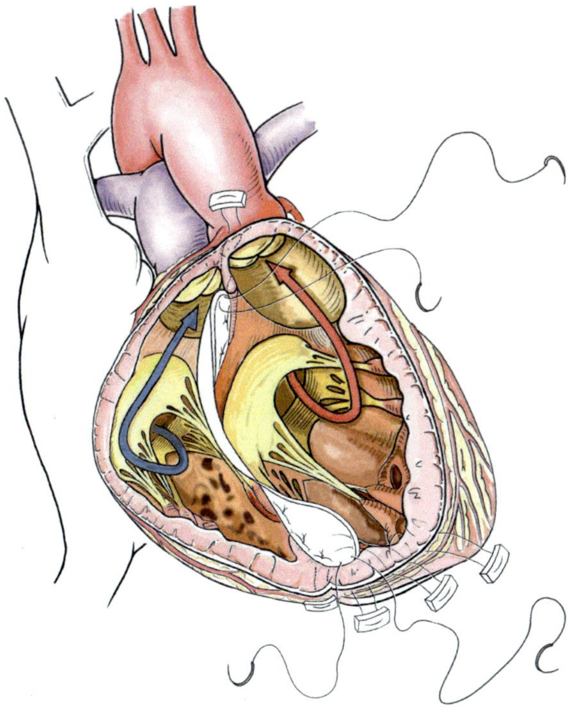

Fig. 3.7 Single ventricular septation surgery: intracardiac blood flow of single ventricle suitable for separation surgery

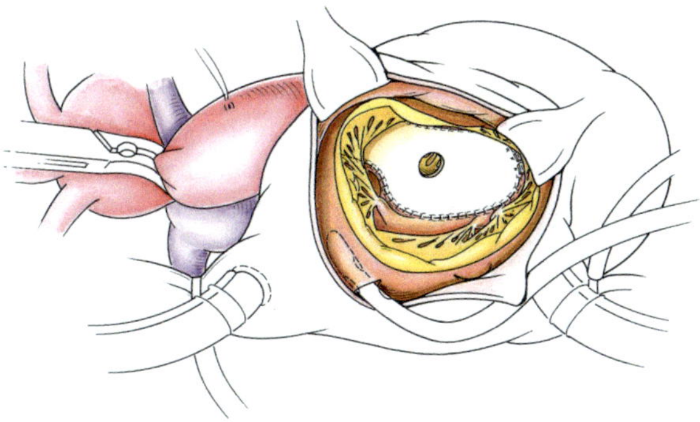

Fig. 3.8 Single ventricular septation surgery: the perforated patch

presented in the region of septation or endocardium as suture points, the patch can also be sutured from the outside to the inside of the heart using an interrupted suture with small pads. Attention should be paid to avoid injury to the coronary arteries when the needle passes through the cardiac muscle (Fig. 3.7).

A small hole of 5–10 mm in diameter left in the patch can balance the arteriovenous blood flow initially after the separation operation; this hole can be closed later by an intervention approach (Fig. 3.8).

Ebert created the two-stage septation surgery in 1984. During the first stage, a small patch was placed at the apex, while another patch was placed between the atrioventricular and semilunar valves, leaving the middle part untouched between

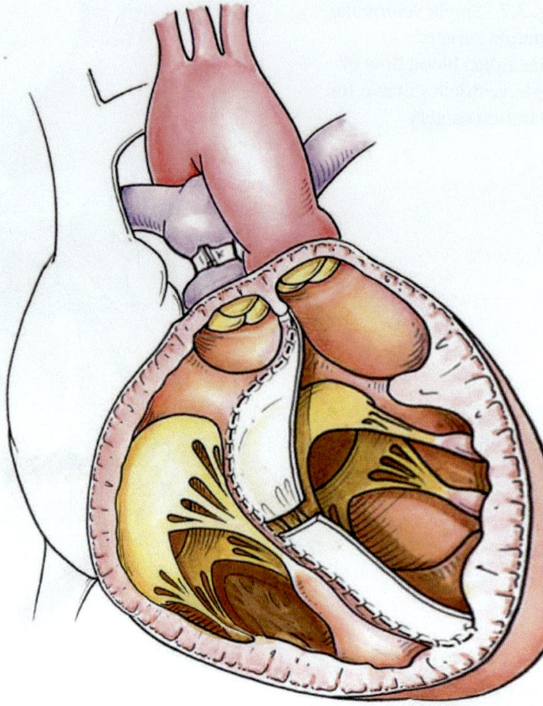

Fig. 3.9 Single ventricular septation surgery: Ebert staging surgery

the two patches. Pulmonary artery banding is performed simultaneously. Stage II of the surgery was performed at 6–18 months after the first stage; the middle part of the ventricular septal defect was oversewn with another patch (Fig. 3.9).

An extracardiac conduit with a valve should be adopted in septation surgeries for cases with pulmonary artery stenosis or postoperative pulmonary artery banding. The septation operation was performed by using a patch with a large hole during the first stage (Fig. 3.10).

In the second surgical stage, the stenotic pulmonary artery is resected and the proximal end is oversewn. Following the opening of the artificially separated small right ventricle as a right ventricular outflow tract, the large hole made on the previous patch is patched (Fig. 3.11).

The pulmonary artery, which is stenotic and unable to form, is replaced by using a valved homograft or xenograft to ensure no pulmonary valve stenosis or regurgitation. Because the separated right ventricle is so small that it can only pump blood in the pulmonary circulation, any additional load will cause the small right ventricle to fail. Because valved homografts and xenografts are difficult to obtain for the main pulmonary artery, extracardiac valved conduits can be used for some older patients, and valved biological vascular grafts of bovine jugular veins can be used for children less than ten years of age. The Contegra graft produced by Medtronic Company, which has received FDA and CE approval, has been used for more than ten years in

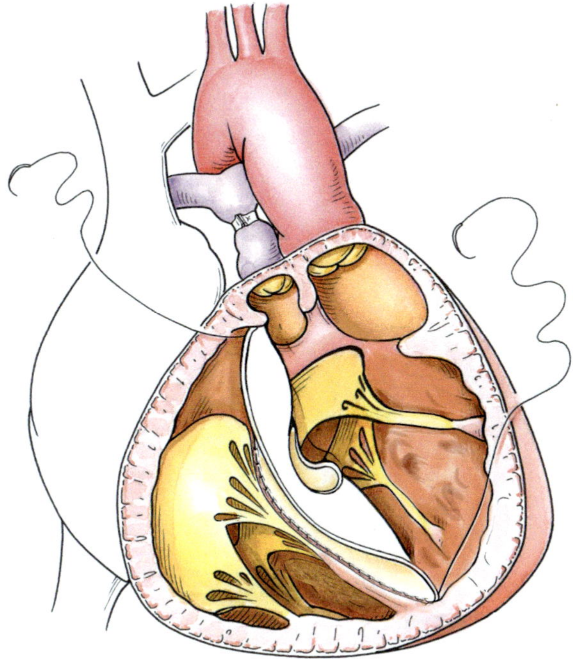

Fig. 3.10 Single ventricular septation surgery: pulmonary artery banding, patch separation

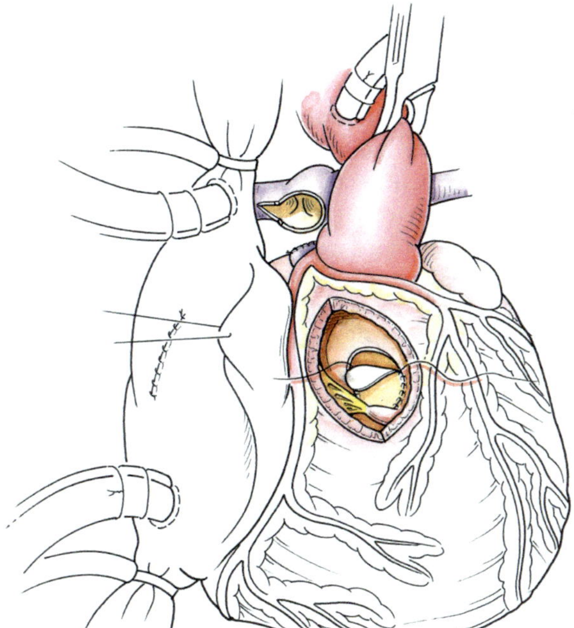

Fig. 3.11 Stage II single ventricular septation surgery: resection of local narrow pulmonary artery, closing reserve hole

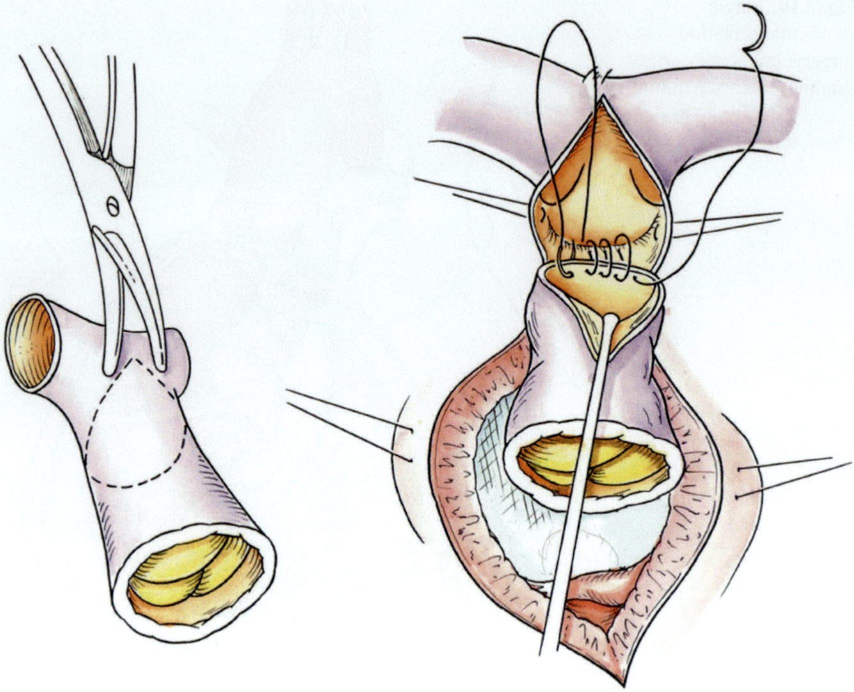

Fig. 3.12 Stage II single ventricular septation surgery: reconstruction with flap grafts of the pulmonary artery and outflow tract

a clinical setting. According to the distance from the pulmonary branches to the right ventricular outflow tract, the valved conduit is trimmed to an appropriate length. Suturing from the rear wall to the front wall of the pulmonary artery is performed first at its distal end, and 5-0 or 6-0 continuous Prolene sutures are generally used according to the age of the child. If the patient has stable perfusion pressure, normal oxygen saturation, normal urine volume, unobstructed venous blood return, little pulmonary blood reflux during CPB, and is without a residual leak in the ventricular septum defect already repaired, the ascending aorta can be opened after left heart air venting. The anastomosis between the pulmonary artery and the outflow tract can be completed under beating conditions (Fig. 3.12).

The concept of absorbable polydioxanone sutures (PDS) can be very attractive to the patient and surgeon due to their advantage of leaving no foreign objects within the tissue after surgery. However, actual clinical results show that tissue responses to PDS absorption lead to much more adjacent tissue adhesion, scarring, and anastomotic stenosis than Prolene, to which the tissues have no response and do not form adhesions.

Fig. 3.13 Stage II single ventricular septation surgery: reconstruction with patch of the right ventricular outflow tract

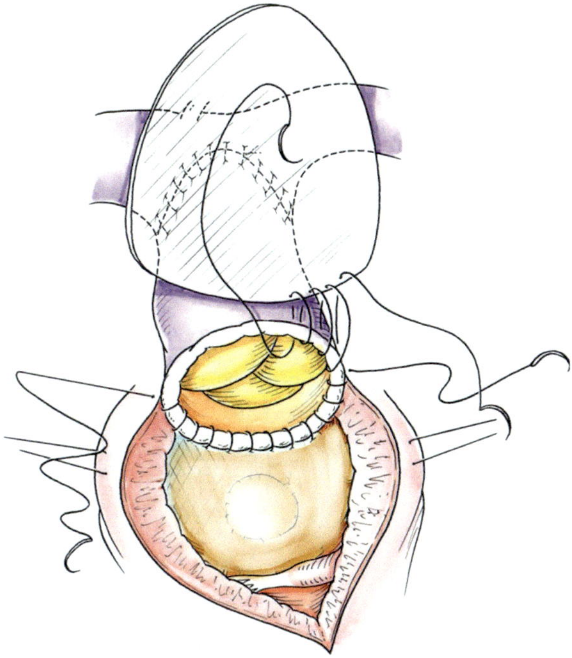

After the distal pulmonary artery anastomosis is complete, the right ventricular outflow tract can next be addressed. In general, it is necessary to form the outflow tract by using polytetrafluoroethylene (Gore-Tex) patches. To form this outflow tract, alternatively, a Gore-Tex conduit can be split and shaped into an arc-like vessel to cover the space between the right ventricular outflow tract and the pulmonary artery grafts. It is recommended to use Prolene for the anastomosis of the posterior wall of the pulmonary graft to the right ventricle and to knot the Prolene at both ends. The patch should be cut according to the size of the curved triangle and stitched onto the right ventricular outflow tract. Another option besides Prolene sutures is to specifically use Gore-Tex sutures. A Gore-Tex suture is compatible with a Gore-Tex patch such that bleeding rarely occurs when tightening the 5-0 suture. However, bleeding occasionally appears at large pinpoints; gauze compression and protamine to neutralize heparin can be helpful in these situations (Fig. 3.13).

Figure 3.14 illustrates the Rastelli surgery (Rastelli et al. 1965), a surgical technique to connect the pulmonary artery that is stenotic but could not be reconstructed and the stenotic outflow tract of right ventricle by using a homograft or xenograft arterial conduit with a valve. The Rastelli surgery put this valved conduit in the right posterior side of the ascending aorta, thereby preventing right ventricular outflow tract and pulmonary artery from being compressed by closed chest after the surgery.

Fig. 3.14 Stage II single ventricular septation surgery: surgery completed

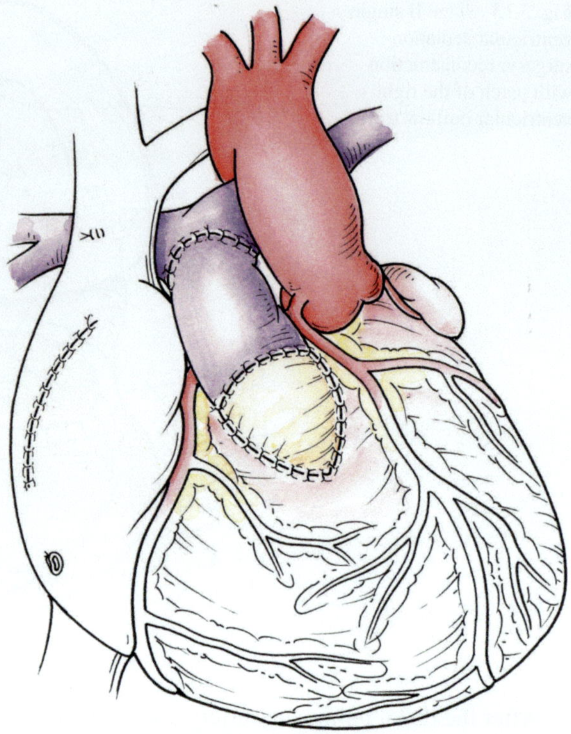

Notes According to the early Van Praagh classification of single ventricle, type IIIA of single ventricle can undergo septation surgery. If the two atrioventricular valves are normal in both function and shape, a small so-called right ventricle can be artificially separated from the single ventricle. Because the aorta lies to the left and in front of the pulmonary artery with the outflow tract directly below the aortic valve, arterial and venous blood flow lines are parallel, and the ventricular septum can be repaired easily. However, the whole operation is very difficult, and postoperative complications and surgical mortality rates are high. When paired with pulmonary artery stenosis, the operative procedure becomes even more difficult. After the development of other surgical methods to treat the single ventricle, especially after the International Congenital Heart Surgery Naming and Database System defined that single ventricles, in principle, cannot be treated with septation surgery, the septation procedure has rarely been performed again. Similar to the cavopulmonary connection operation, in principle, the septation surgery is used to separate arterial and venous blood flow, and resultantly reduce the burden of the single ventricle. The most successful surgeries show that the life quality and long-term survival rate of patients who have undergone septation surgery are better than that of cavopulmonary connection surgery patients. Reconsideration of septation surgery may provide a novel concept for the surgical treatment of functional single ventricle.

References

Ebert PA. Staged partitioning of single ventricle. J Thorac Cardiovasc Surg. 1984;88(6):908–13.

Rastelli GC, Ongley PA, Davis GD, Kirklin JW. Surgical repair for pulmonary valve atresia with coronary-pulmonary artery fistula: report of case. Mayo Clin Proc. 1965;40:521–7.

Van Praagh R. Segmental approach to diagnosis. In: Nadas' pediatric cardiology. Philadelphia: Hanley & Belfus; 1992. p. 27–35.

Chapter 4
Classic Glenn Surgery: Early Palliative Surgery

Bin Qiao and Meng Zhu

Carlon et al. in 1951 and Glenn and Patiño in 1954 explored in their experimental work the feasibility of a connection between the superior vena cava (SVC) and the pulmonary artery to increase pulmonary blood flow (Glenn and Patiño 1954). In 1958, Professor Glenn at Yale University reported the first clinical case with this principle applied (Glenn 1958).

Since the late 1950s, the Glenn shunt has been used as an anastomosis of the superior vena cava to the right pulmonary artery (RPA) for the treatment of different cyanotic congenital heart diseases in order to improve pulmonary blood flow. Unlike systemic to pulmonary artery shunts, the Glenn shunt would not cause ventricular volume overload or increase ventricular work (Jacobs et al. 1996). The Glenn shunt allows venous blood to be further oxygenated in the lungs rather than in an arterio-venous mixture, provides a low systemic venous pressure, and no risk of increasing pulmonary vascular resistance (PVR) (Bridges et al. 1990; Hopkins et al. 1985). The Glenn shunt is a palliative instead of corrective surgery to treat cardiac malformations.

In the past, the Glenn shunt has been regarded as one of the operative approaches to palliate cyanotic congenital heart disease with only a unidirectional shunt between the superior vena cava and the right pulmonary artery. In recent years, this method has been modified and transformed into an end-to-side anastomosis between the superior vena cava and pulmonary artery in which the superior vena cava blood flows toward both the left and right pulmonary arteries simultaneously. It can act to

B. Qiao (✉)
Cardiovascular Institute, General Hospital of Jinan Military Region, Jinan, China

Cardiac Surgery Center, Western District of Shandong Provincial Hospital, Jinan, China

M. Zhu
Institute of Cardiovascular Diseases, Jinan Military Region General Hospital of PLA, Jinan, China

B. Qiao et al. (eds.), *Surgical Atlas of Functional Single Ventricle and Hypoplastic Left Heart Syndrome*, https://doi.org/10.1007/978-981-10-8435-5_4

mediate surgery for further correction operations or for a total cavopulmonary connection Fontan surgery. The former is now referred to as the classical Glenn shunt, while the latter is called a bidirectional Glenn shunt.

The classical Glenn shunt can be performed without cardiopulmonary bypass. The superior vena cava and the right pulmonary artery were exposed following a median sternotomy and pericardium suspension. The best position to transecting the superior vena cava is in the conjunction between the superior vena cava and right atrium, about 1 cm away from the sinoatrial node (Fig. 4.1).

The distal end of the right pulmonary artery can be revealed by cutting open the pleura at the right hilar. With a small cotton ball, the upper, middle, and lower lobes of right pulmonary artery are dissected bluntly. Two laps of a thin rubber band are placed across them respectively to prevent the return of blood when the anastomosis is performed. The azygos vein, frequently at the posterior side of the superior vena cava, is oversewn or ligated away from the superior vena cava as far as possible. The dotted line shows the transection site of the azygos vein on the superior vena cava. The ascending aorta is pulled out with a retractor to expose the proximal right pulmonary artery, which can then be ligated. Ensure that the phrenic nerve is not damaged during the entire operative procedure (Fig. 4.2).

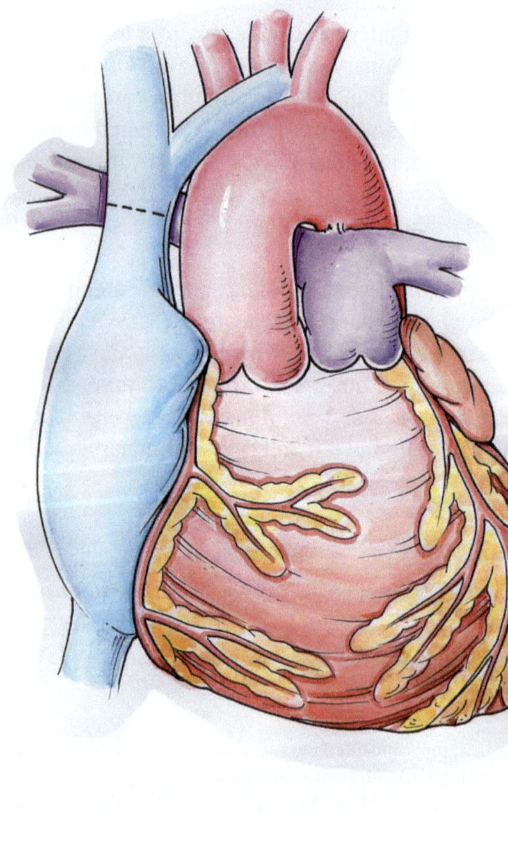

Fig. 4.1 Classic Glenn shunt: the position of transecting superior vena cava

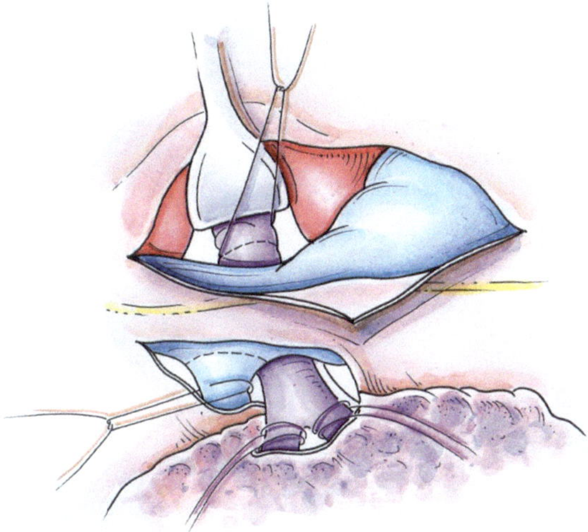

Fig. 4.2 Classic Glenn shunt: suturing and ligating azygos vein and the proximal part of right pulmonary artery

Since this surgery does not require cardiopulmonary bypass, the clamping time of the superior vena cava and the right pulmonary artery should be short. Cyanotic patients often have a certain tolerance of cyanosis. This surgery can be performed with anesthesia, intubation, and high concentrations of oxygen inhalation under different circumstances. The classical Glenn shunt begins with a transection of the right pulmonary artery. Heparin is applied before blocking the right pulmonary artery at a dose of 150 unit/kg for a child and 500–10,000 unit/kg for an adult. Heparin can be neutralized by an appropriate protamine dosage according to the ACT condition if there is no bleeding after the surgery. Postoperative anticoagulation is not necessary due to the lack of foreign body implantation. A high concentration of oxygen inhalation was served through the left lung ventilation. The operation is started by traversing the right pulmonary artery. After the cardiac end of the right pulmonary artery has been ligated, and the right, middle, and lower lobes of the pulmonary artery have also been respectively blocked, the right pulmonary artery is transected, maintaining a proper length that ensures a tension-free anastomosis with the superior vena cava. The superior vena cava is transected 1 cm above its junction with the right atrium following the blockage of its distal and proximal ends with a noninvasive vascular clamp. The atrial end of the superior vena cava can be oversewn with 5 or 6-0 Prolene, and its distal end is later anastomosed to the right pulmonary artery (Fig. 4.3).

The key of the classic Glenn shunt is to avoid the tension at the anastomosis between superior vena cava and the right pulmonary artery, as well as to avoid anastomotic stenosis caused by human factors. To do this, for example, the cavopulmonary anastomosis should be large enough and the Prolene sutures should be small, using 6-0 sutures for a small child. Although finer continuous sutures for a child would be partially broken during his growth due to intravascular pressure, this factor does not usually cause the anastomosis to relatively narrow. Anastomotic stenosis can also be technically avoided by the use of continuous sutures for the posterior

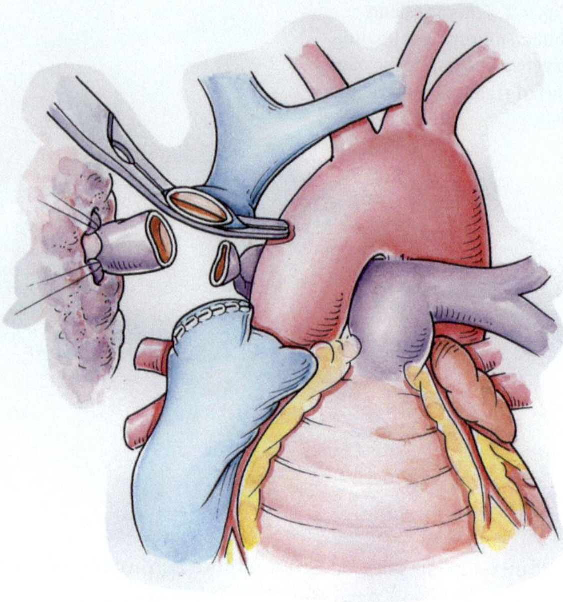

Fig. 4.3 Classic Glenn shunt: transection of right pulmonary artery, superior vena cava

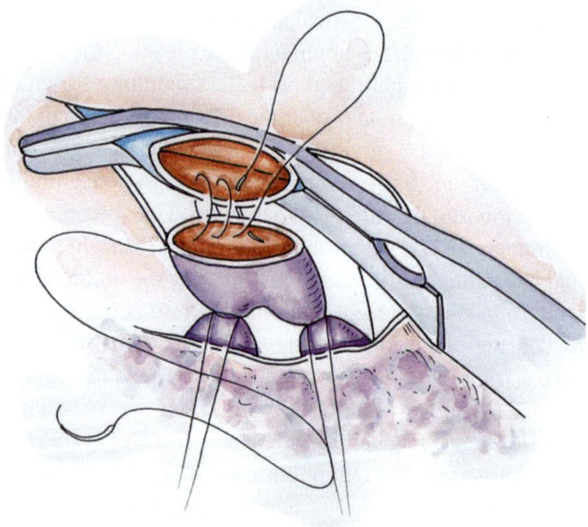

Fig. 4.4 Classic Glenn shunt: superior vena cava and right pulmonary artery anastomosis

wall and interrupted sutures for the anterior wall. For PDS absorbable sutures, tissue reaction to their absorption can cause local tissue scarring and resulting anastomotic narrowing. Based on this reaction, the author does not recommend the application of PDS sutures for such an anastomosis (Fig. 4.4).

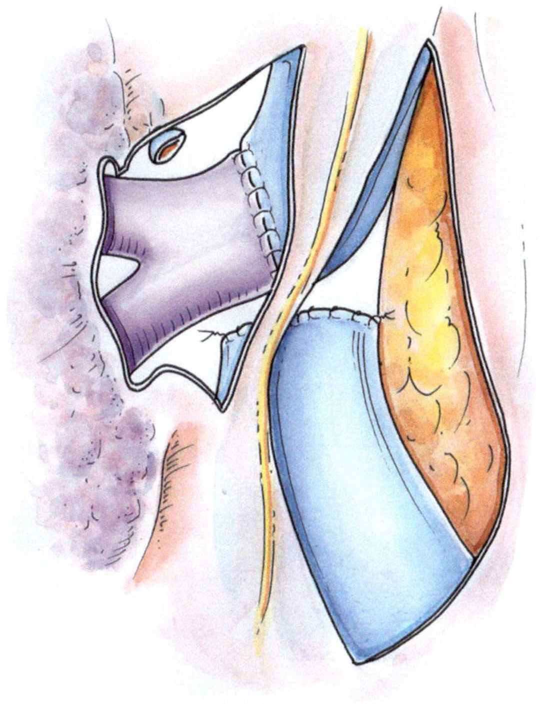

Fig. 4.5 Classic Glenn shunt: superior vena cava and right pulmonary artery anastomosis completed

After the anastomosis of the superior vena cava to the right pulmonary artery has been completed (Fig. 4.5), the blockage of the distal ends of the right pulmonary artery and superior vena cava can be released. Without significant bleeding observed at the anastomosis, suction and lung expansion can be done via tracheal cannula. The increase of lung capacity can cause a negative pressure in lungs. This negative pressure could help the venous blood, which was stagnated in the head and the upper body, quickly flow into the right pulmonary artery. Heparin can be excreted automatically as long as the ACT value is not high.

Figure 4.6 shows a final Classic Glenn shunt. After the classical Glenn shunt surgery, oxygen saturation will quickly rise. The pleura can be opened for the placement of a chest tube. With the upper part of the pericardial cavity closed, its lower part is open for the routine placement of two pericardial drainage tubes. This operation is limited to the scope of the right upper chest with less cardiopulmonary operating, so it does not require a thorough exposure and double-lumen endotracheal intubation.

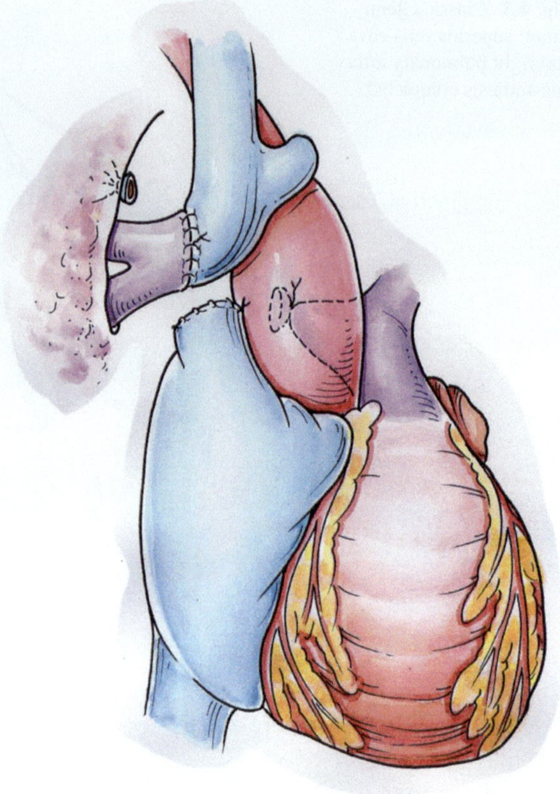

Fig. 4.6 Classic Glenn shunt: surgery completed

Notes The classic Glenn shunt was applied for most of the cases of tricuspid valve atresia or single ventricle in the 1960s and 1970s. With other corrective operations for functional single ventricle having since been carried out, different cavopulmonary connection modes have appeared, such as the modified bidirectional Glenn shunt and total cavopulmonary connection Fontan surgery. Since the development of these modes, the simple classical Glenn shunt surgery has rarely been applied. For some cases with functional single ventricle who have undergone the classical Glenn shunt surgery, in fact, the Fontan surgery with a connection between the inferior vena cava and left pulmonary artery can still be implemented in later time. However, this type of reoperation could not have been continued in those past years because of the lack of reoperation and cardiopulmonary bypass experience, as well as the requirement of extensive mobilization of large vessels such as the pulmonary artery. Today, the total cavopulmonary connection has been standardized, and the modified bidirectional Glenn shunt has become an intermediate surgery before final operations on functional single ventricle.

References

Bridges ND, Jonas RA, Mayer JE, Flanagan MF, Keane JF, Castaneda AR. Bidirectional cavopulmonary anastomosis as interim palliation for high-risk Fontan candidates. Early results. Circulation. 1990;82(5 Suppl):IV170–6.

Glenn WWL. Circulatory bypass of the right side of the heart. N Engl J Med. 1958;259(3):117–20. https://doi.org/10.1056/nejm195807172590304.

Glenn WWL, Patiño JF. Circulatory by-pass of the right heart. I. Preliminary observations on the direct delivery of vena caval blood into the pulmonary arterial circulation. Azygos vein-pulmonary artery shunt. Yale J Biol Med. 1954;27(3):147–51.

Hopkins RA, Armstrong BE, Serwer GA, Peterson RJ, Oldham HN. Physiological rationale for a bidirectional cavopulmonary shunt. A versatile complement to the Fontan principle. J Thorac Cardiovasc Surg. 1985;90(3):391–8.

Jacobs ML, Rychik J, Rome JJ, Apostolopoulou S, Pizarro C, Murphy JD, Norwood WI. Early reduction of the volume work of the single ventricle: The hemi-fontan operation. Ann Thorac Surg. 1996;62(2):456–62. https://doi.org/10.1016/0003-4975(96)00279-2.

Chapter 5
Bidirectional Glenn Shunt: Stage I Palliative Surgery

Bin Qiao and Ji Feng Ju

Classical Glenn surgery is simple with a low mortality rate, after which patient cyanosis is alleviated and symptoms are improved significantly. In the 1960s and early 1970s, classical Glenn surgery was widely used to treat tricuspid valve atresia with good short-term outcomes. However, most of the patients once again developed cyanosis. Based on the Haller's study on animals, Dogliotti et al had made some improvements on classical Glenn surgery, including transecting the superior vena cava, closing its atrial end and anastomosing its distal end end-to-side to the right pulmonary artery. These improvements ensure not only continuity between the pulmonary artery and the superior vena cava, but also blood flow to the bilateral pulmonary artery. The bidirectional Glenn shunt, hence its name, was widely used in the clinic for the treatment of functional single ventricle as a better surgical alternative to the classical Glenn shunt, and later became an intermediate surgery for the total cavopulmonary connection of the Fontan operation (Hopkins et al. 1985; Mazzera et al. 1989).

General anesthesia and tracheal intubation followed by blockage of the superior vena cava or right pulmonary artery cannot guarantee ideal oxygen saturation for a child with severe cyanosis. Cardiopulmonary bypass can be performed under normal temperature without blockage of the ascending aorta, such that the operation can be complemented under beating-heart conditions. Of course, the cannulation position of the superior vena cava should be higher to facilitate the end-to-side anastomosis of the superior vena cava to the right pulmonary artery. Above 1 cm of its

B. Qiao (✉)
Cardiovascular Institute, General Hospital of Jinan Military Region, Jinan, China

Cardiac Surgery Center, Western District of Shandong Provincial Hospital, Jinan, China

J. F. Ju
Institute of Cardiovascular Diseases, Jinan Military Region General Hospital of PLA, Jinan, China

B. Qiao et al. (eds.), *Surgical Atlas of Functional Single Ventricle and Hypoplastic Left Heart Syndrome*, https://doi.org/10.1007/978-981-10-8435-5_5

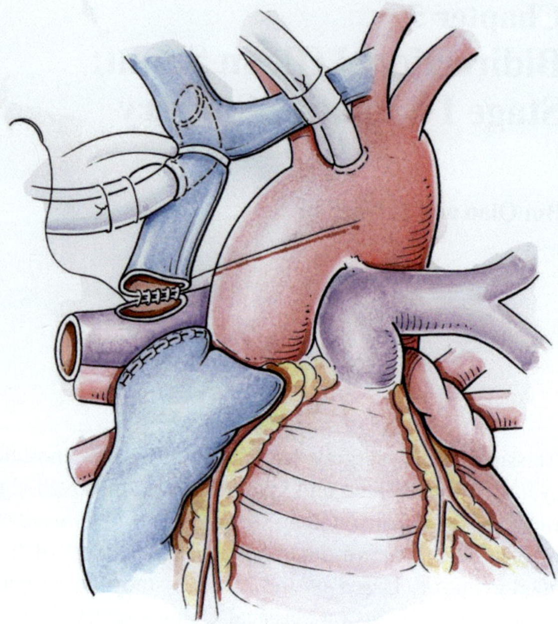

Fig. 5.1 Bidirectional Glenn shunt: end-to-side anastomosis of superior vena cava and right pulmonary artery under cardiopulmonary bypass

junction with the right atrium where it is far away from the sinoatrial node, the superior vena cava can be transected after its cannula sleeve is tightened. The right pulmonary artery is incised at the corresponding position on its superior surface. Pulmonary blood return should not be extensive if inferior and superior vena cava drainage is satisfied; otherwise, the right pulmonary artery should be partially blocked to facilitate the suturing of the superior vena cava to the pulmonary artery. Continuous 6-0 Prolene sutures are used from the anastomosis posterior wall to its anterior wall where knots are tied (Fig. 5.1).

In general, the hypoxia tolerance ability of patients with a higher hemoglobin level is stronger than in patients with a normal one. Given general anesthesia with total oxygen ventilation, cardiopulmonary bypass is not needed in the bidirectional Glenn procedure. Under these circumstances, the divided superior vena cava should be blocked by an occlusion clamp and the right pulmonary artery should also be blocked by a sidewalls occlusion clamp (Fig. 5.2). The end-to-side anastomosis method should be interpreted as described above.

After completion of the bidirectional Glenn shunt, the blood from the superior vena cava flows toward both the left and right pulmonary arteries. It has replaced the classical Glenn shunt (Fig. 5.3).

The left superior vena cava (LSVC), if presented, must be divided and end-to-side anastomosed to the left pulmonary artery. It is generally a presentation of a left superior vena cava that the right superior vena cava (RSVC) is found to be relatively small after thoracotomy. Dissection of the left superior vena cava sometimes requires flipping of the heart, so the surgery is better performed under cardiopulmonary bypass also without ascending aorta blockage, with the heart beating. To ensure

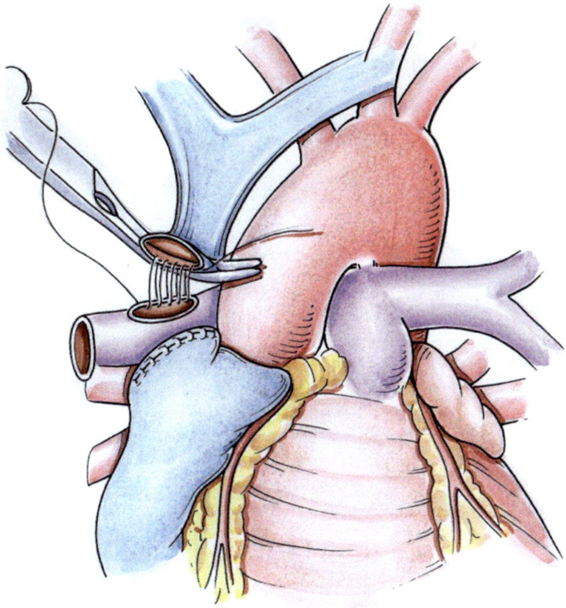

Fig. 5.2 Bidirectional Glenn shunt: end-to-side anastomosis of superior vena cava and right pulmonary artery without cardiopulmonary bypass

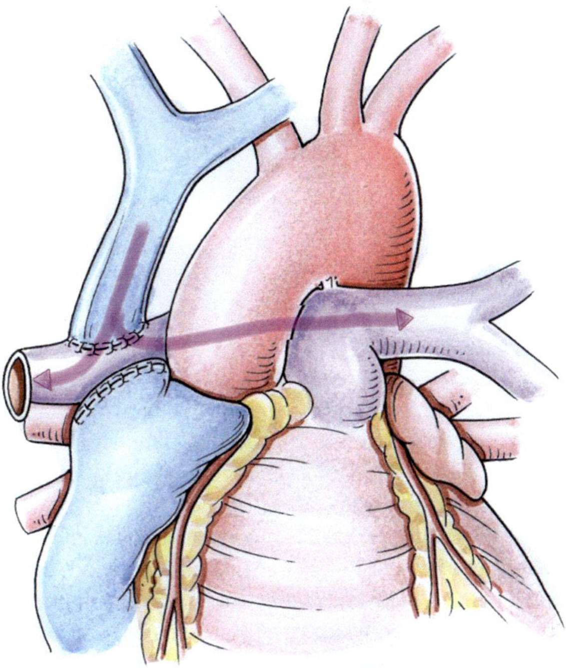

Fig. 5.3 Bidirectional Glenn shunt: blood flow in superior vena cava

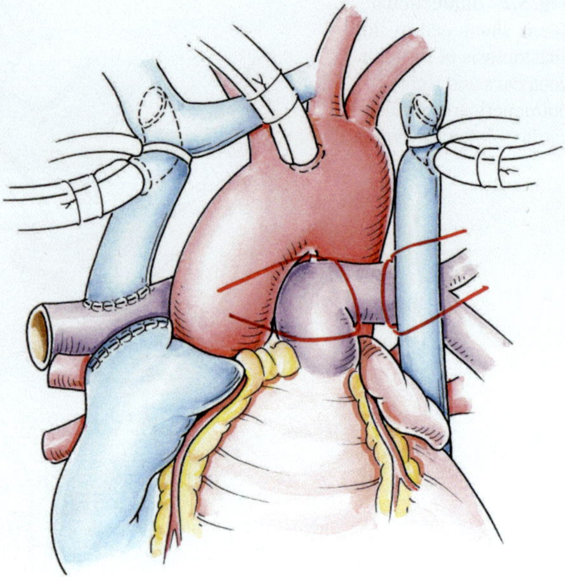

Fig. 5.4 Bilateral bidirectional Glenn shunt: cannula in left superior vena cava

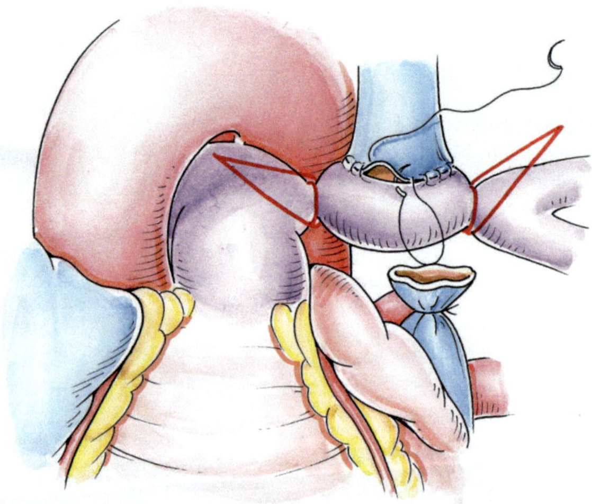

Fig. 5.5 Bilateral bidirectional Glenn shunt: end-to-side anastomosis of left superior vena cava and left pulmonary artery

a fully venous blood return of cardiopulmonary bypass and to facilitate the anastomosis of the left superior vena cava to the left pulmonary artery, a cannula is placed in the left superior vena cava (Fig. 5.4).

The superior vena cava is reopened after completion of the right sided end-to-side cavopulmonary anastomosis. At its proximal end, the left superior vena cava is dissected free, divided, and oversewn. Following blockage of the pulmonary artery with a rubber band in both sides of the anastomosis, an end-to-side anastomosis of the left superior vena cava to the left pulmonary artery is performed following the creation of an incision at an appropriate location on the left pulmonary artery (Fig. 5.5).

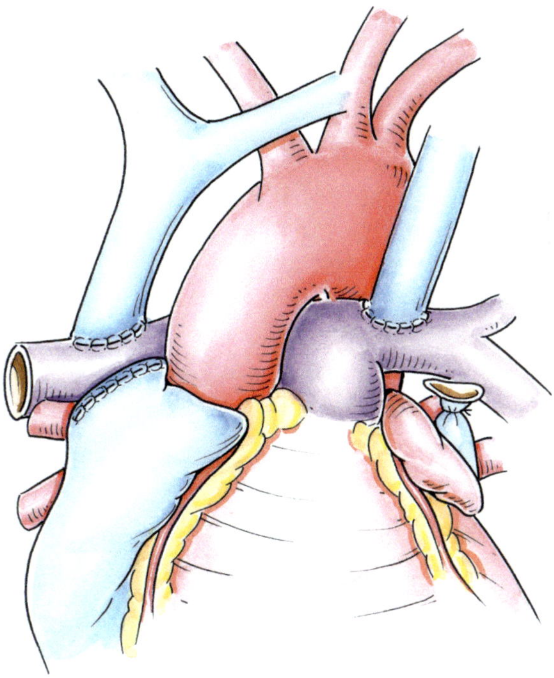

Fig. 5.6 Bilateral bidirectional Glenn shunt: anastomosis completed

For cases with a persistent left superior vena cava (PLSVC), the connection between the left superior vena cava and left pulmonary artery should be undertaken at the same time to ensure that the vena cava blood returns fully into the pulmonary circulation (Fig. 5.6).

References

Hopkins RA, Armstrong BE, Serwer GA, Peterson RJ, Oldham HN. Physiological rationale for a bidirectional cavopulmonary shunt. A versatile complement to the Fontan principle. J Thorac Cardiovasc Surg. 1985;90(3):391–8.

Mazzera E, Corno A, Picardo S, Di Donato R, Marino B, Costa D, Marcelletti C. Bidirectional cavopulmonary shunts: clinical applications as staged or definitive palliation. Ann Thorac Surg. 1989;47(3):415–20. https://doi.org/10.1016/0003-4975(89)90384-6.

Chapter 6
Qiao's Surgery: Qiao's Modified Bidirectional Glenn Shunt and Incomplete Fontan Surgery

Bin Qiao and Tong Jian Wang

6.1 Qiao's Modified Bidirectional Glenn Shunt

Qiao's surgery includes two surgical methods. One is Qiao's modified bidirectional Glenn shunt; the other is incomplete Fontan surgery, i.e., Qiao's preservation of pulsating forward blood Flow. In Qiao's modified bidirectional Glenn shunt, the superior vena cava is anastomosed to the right pulmonary artery, while the divided innominate vein (INV) is anastomosed to the left pulmonary artery; the size of the anastomosis matches the superior vena cava and innominate vein in diameter. The modified approach has advantages in relation to the traditional bidirectional Glenn shunt in that the anastomosis is significantly enlarged and the pulmonary blood flow distribution to both lungs is more reasonable. It could potentially be adopted as the first stage palliation for subsequent staged Fontan surgeries.

The patient is placed supine. A standard median sternotomy approach is employed. The thymus is subtotally resected. The pericardium is opened longitudinally to expose the heart and supported with stay sutures. The innominate vein, superior vena cava, azygos vein, and left pulmonary artery are all dissected fully. The azygos vein is ligated and excised. Cardiopulmonary bypass is commenced following necessary intubation. The drainage cannula of the superior vena cava is placed in the junction of the superior vena cava and innominate vein (Fig. 6.1).

The superior vena cava is divided at about 5mm above its junction with the right atrium. Its cardiac end is oversewn and its distal end is end-to-side anastomosed to

B. Qiao (✉)
Cardiovascular Institute, General Hospital of Jinan Military Region, Jinan, China

Cardiac Surgery Center, Western District of Shandong Provincial Hospital, Jinan, China

T. J. Wang
Institute of Cardiovascular Diseases, Jinan Military Region General Hospital of PLA, Jinan, China

B. Qiao et al. (eds.), *Surgical Atlas of Functional Single Ventricle and Hypoplastic Left Heart Syndrome*, https://doi.org/10.1007/978-981-10-8435-5_6

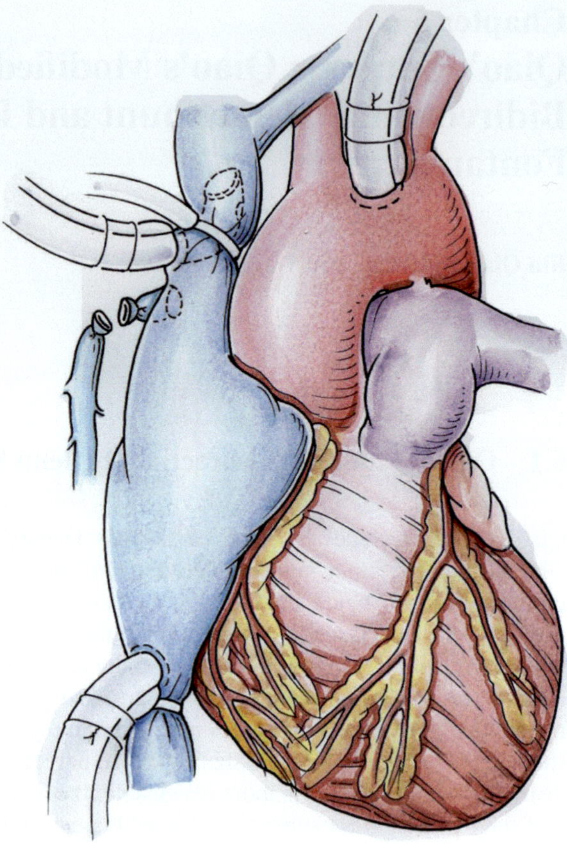

Fig. 6.1 Qiao's modified bidirectional Glenn shunt: ligating and cutting azygos vein

the longitudinal incision on the anterior surface of the right pulmonary artery with 7-0 new-style absorbable PDS (Polydioxanone) (Fig. 6.2). During the time in which the new absorbable suture is absorbed, tissue reactions are too small to cause any significant anastomotic stenosis, as was the case with past PDS sutures.

The innominate vein is divided at its junction with the superior vena cava and the resulting incision on the superior vena cava is oversewn with continuous Prolene. It is sufficient to remain 5mm of the innominate vein stump. Too short a stump can lead to superior vena cava stenosis as the incision is sewn up. On the contrary, too long a stump might lead to thrombosis, or even to a failed anastomosis procedure (Fig. 6.3).

An end-to-side anastomosis is performed between the divided innominate vein and a longitudinal incision of the left pulmonary artery. The back wall of the anastomosis is first sutured anteriorly to its front wall, followed by knotting. The main pulmonary artery is divided and then closed with continuous sutures (Fig. 6.4).

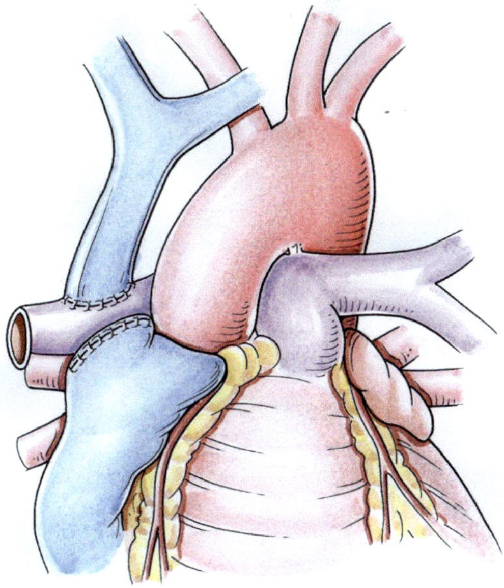

Fig. 6.2 Qiao's modified bidirectional Glenn shunt: end-to-side anastomosis of superior vena cava and right pulmonary artery

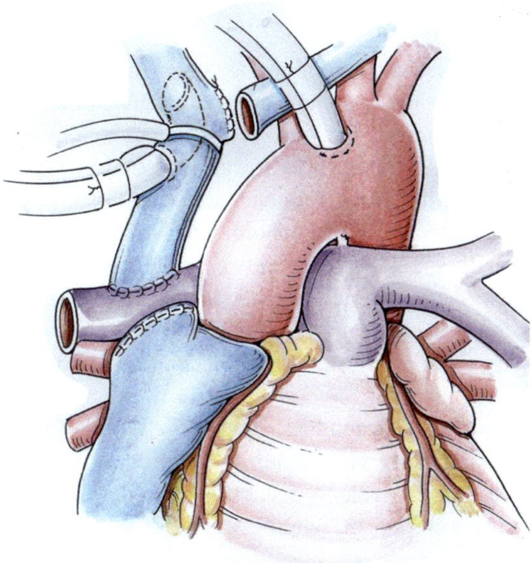

Fig. 6.3 Qiao's modified bidirectional Glenn shunt: transection site on innominate vein

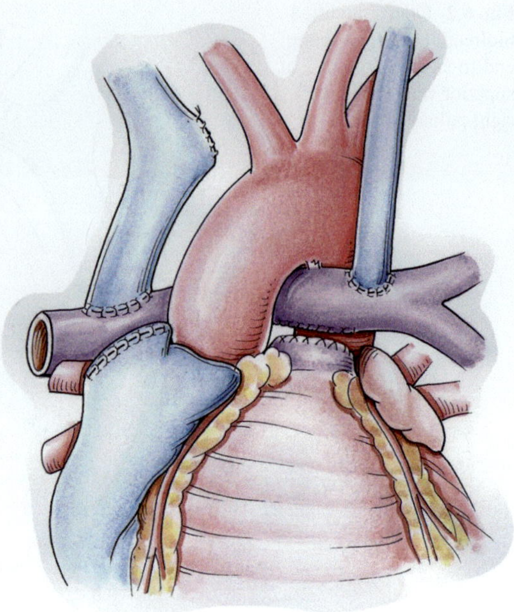

Fig. 6.4 Qiao's modified bidirectional Glenn shunt: end-to-side anastomosis of innominate vein and left pulmonary artery, cutting and ligating main pulmonary artery

6.2 Incomplete Fontan Surgery: Qiao's Preservation of Pulsating Forward Blood Flow

Fontan surgery is defined as a total cavopulmonary connection which completely separates the systemic and pulmonary circulations. In intra-atrial lateral tunnel Fontan surgery, the atrial septal defect is not completely closed, and the lateral tunnel is fenestrated. In extracardiac conduit Fontan surgery, a fenestration is made between the extracardiac conduit and the adjacent atrium by direct fashion or with artificial vasculature. Incomplete Fontan surgery refers to the operation that intentionally creates a shunt between the systemic and pulmonary circulations. Because pulmonary vascular resistance may be transiently increased during early Fontan surgery, a shunt is also established at the atrial level during incomplete Fontan surgery to relieve systemic venous pressure and to improve the single ventricle filling.

A pulsating forward blood flow is preserved in Qiao's modified bidirectional Glenn shunt to conduct some of the blood of the inferior vena cava back to the pulmonary artery via the narrow pulmonary valve by the power of ventricular pulsation. It is possible to make this procedure a final palliative approach for functional single ventricles. The procedure can also be called an incomplete Fontan surgery.

The incomplete Fontan surgery can be used to treat the cases with high-risk factors related to Fontan surgery or for those who cannot endure Fontan surgery. Good examples of high-risk factors include >20 mmHg of mean pressure at pulmonary artery and >4 Wood units/m^2 pulmonary vascular resistance index (PVRI). This procedure can reduce the incidence of serious complications that may result from Fontan surgery as the next step, and its long-term effects are not worse when compared to the total cavopulmonary connection. The surgery consists of three main technical points: (1) The main pulmonary artery is longitudinally incised along the middle of its most superior surface, extending inferiorly to a site 1 cm away above the pulmonary valve orifice. The resulting incisions are sutured along the left and right pulmonary arteries with a patch. Subsequently, the left and right pulmonary arteries are relatively extended. The mixed blood in the inferior vena cava is immediately conducted into the shaped left and right pulmonary arteries via the pulmonary valve orifice, and a balanced distribution of bilateral pulmonary blood can therefore be achieved. In addition, extended left and right pulmonary artery can weaken the high-speed impact of anterior pulmonary blood flow to the superior vena cava flow. (2) Another point pertains to probing and dealing with the pulmonary valve orifice. When the valve orifice is larger, the leaflet junction is sutured appropriately; if smaller, it is cut open appropriately. The long-term follow-up of the bidirectional Glenn shunt surgery shows that the valve orifice should not be more than 5mm in diameter. (3) After the innominate vein is divided from the superior vena cava, the superior vena cava is anastomosed to the right pulmonary artery, and the innominate vein is anastomosed to the left pulmonary artery.

This Figure 6.5 shows a functional single ventricle with right ventricular hypoplasia, an anteroposterior atrium, the aorta located in front of the right pulmonary artery, and pulmonary artery stenosis. The dashed line shows the division site of the innominate vein and the incision of the main pulmonary artery.

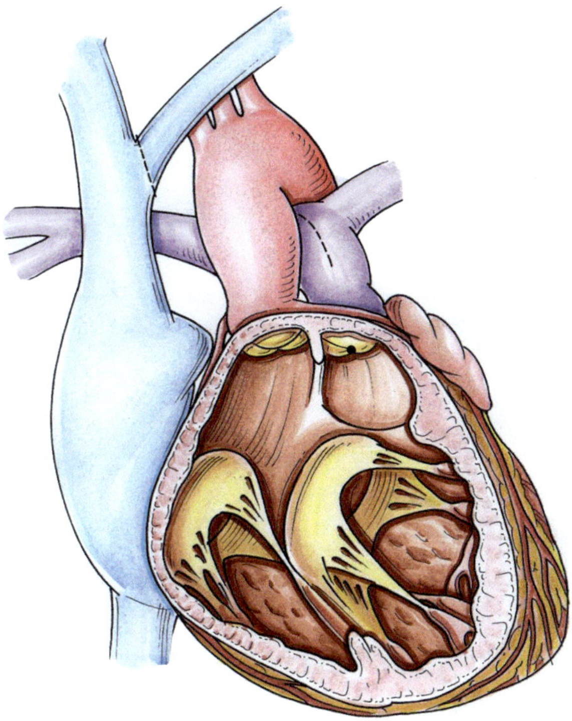

Fig. 6.5 Qiao's incomplete Fontan surgery: innominate vein transection, incision site of main pulmonary artery

Along the bifurcation of the left and right pulmonary arteries, the main pulmonary artery is longitudinally incised and the incision is extended to the site 1 cm away above the pulmonary valve orifice (Fig. 6.6).

The pulmonary valve orifice can be explored and treated through the main pulmonary artery longitudinal incision. When the pulmonary valve orifice is larger, the junction of valve leaflets should be sutured appropriately, maintaining the orifice about 5mm in diameter (Fig. 6.7).

If the pulmonary valve presents stenosis, it should be properly enlarged (Fig. 6.8).

Along the left and right pulmonary arteries, the resulting incision of the main pulmonary artery is supplemented with a patch to ensure that the left and right pulmonary artery branch can be extended to a site 1cm away from the opening of the pulmonary artery valve, and that the main pulmonary artery is shortened accordingly (Fig. 6.9).

Fig. 6.6 Qiao's incomplete Fontan surgery: longitudinal incision on main pulmonary artery

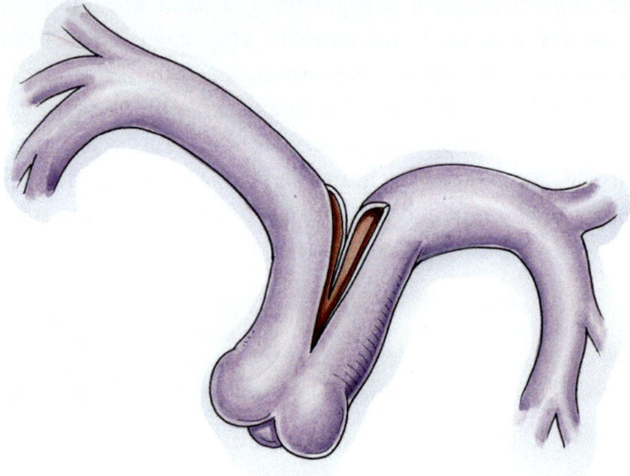

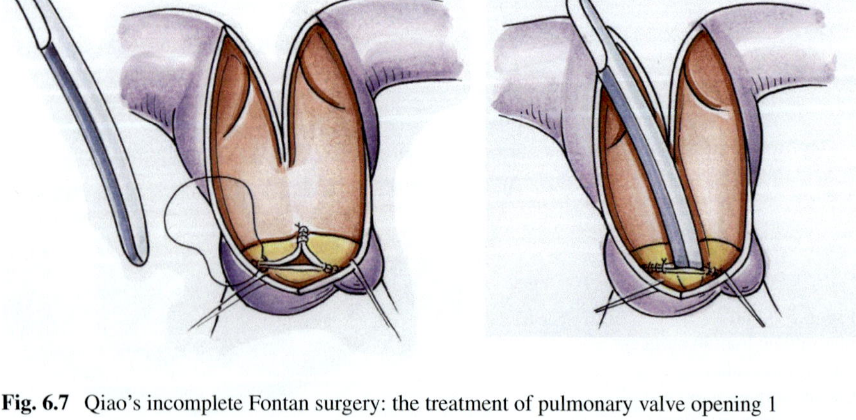

Fig. 6.7 Qiao's incomplete Fontan surgery: the treatment of pulmonary valve opening 1

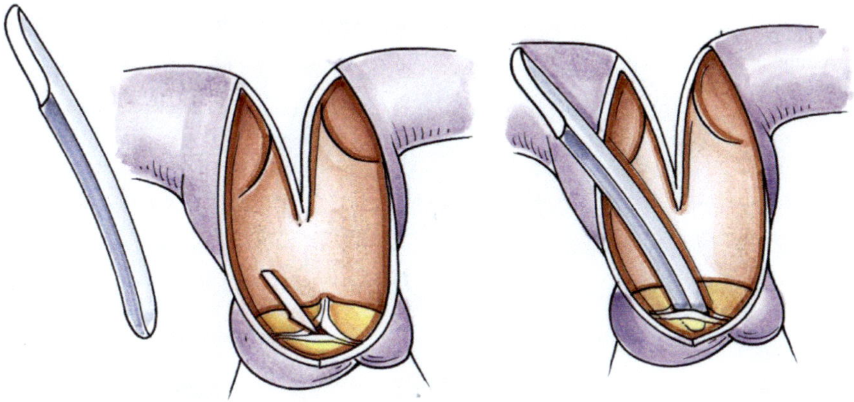

Fig. 6.8 Qiao's incomplete Fontan surgery: the treatment of pulmonary valve opening 2

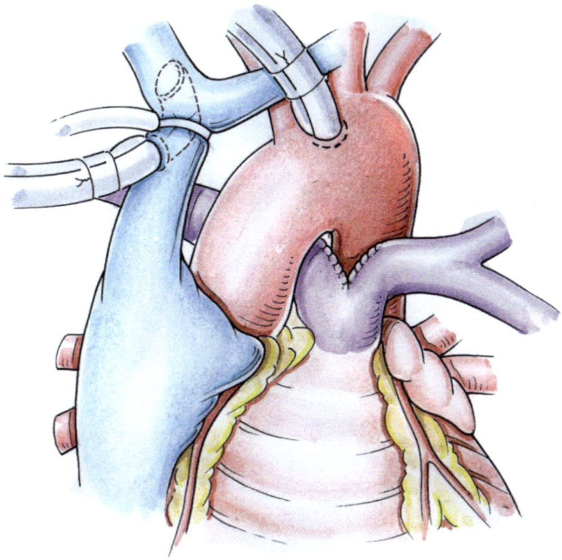

Fig. 6.9 Qiao's incomplete Fontan surgery: suturing main pulmonary artery incision

About 5mm above its junction with the right atrium, the superior vena cava is divided. Its cardiac end is oversewn, and its distal end is end-to-side anastomosed to the longitudinal incision on the anterior surface of the right pulmonary artery with 7-0 new-style absorbable PDS (Polydioxanone) (Fig. 6.10). The way of the anastomosis of innominate vein and left pulmonary artery is same as that in Qiao's modified bidirectional Glenn shunt.

In Qiao's modified bidirectional Glenn surgery maintaining forward pulsatile blood flow, the blood of the superior vena cava subtotally flows into the right lung, the innominate vein blood subtotally flows into the left lung, and the blood mixed through the pulmonary artery valve area flows into the left and right pulmonary arteries in a balanced fashion (Fig. 6.11).

Fig. 6.10 Qiao's incomplete Fontan surgery: cavopulmonary end-to-side anastomosis

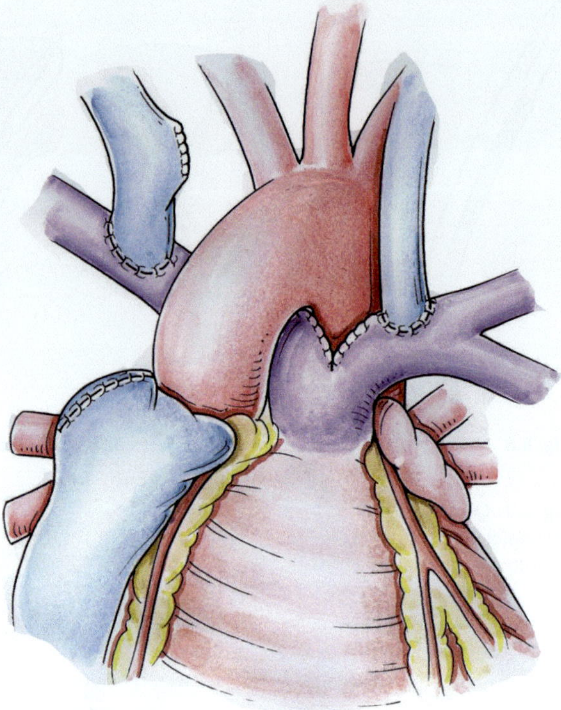

Fig. 6.11 Qiao's incomplete Fontan surgery: blood flow pattern

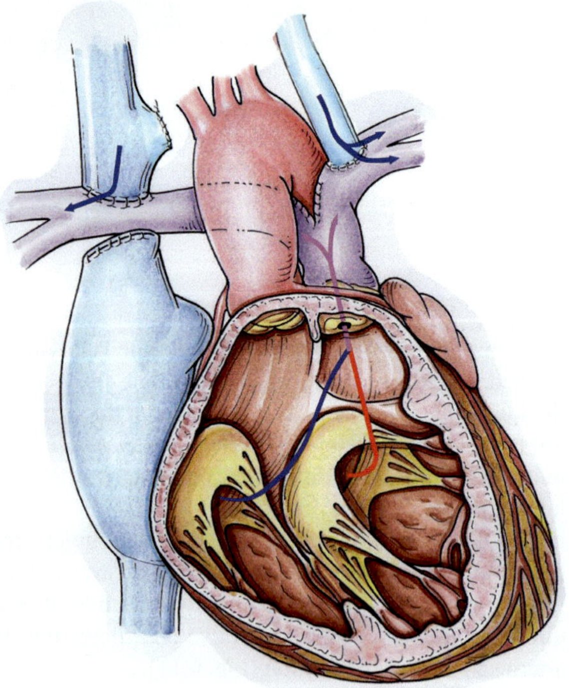

Chapter 7
The Basic Concepts of Traditional Fontan Surgery: Systemic and Pulmonary Circulation Shunt

Bin Qiao and Hai Jie Li

7.1 History of Surgery

In the late 1940s, laboratory studies showed that systemic venous pressure can provide sufficient power to allow venous blood to enter the pulmonary circulation. For the next 10 years, long-term results on a number of animal experiments reported the connection between the superior or inferior vena cava and the right pulmonary artery. In 1951, Carbon suggested that a single left ventricle in some cases with tricuspid valve atresia could sustain two circulations because pulmonary arterial resistance was low. In 1958, Glenn successfully performed the first case of superior vena cava to right pulmonary artery anastomosis to treat a 7-year-old patient who suffered from functional single ventricle with aortic and pulmonary artery stenosis and translocation. This type of end-to-end connection of the superior vena cava to the right pulmonary artery is also known as classical Glenn shunt. In 1966, Haller and his colleagues modified the classic Glenn surgery and performed the anastomosis of the superior vena cava to the pulmonary artery in a dog in which the blood from the superior vena cava flowed into both the left and right pulmonary arteries (Haller et al. 1966). This procedure is now called the bidirectional Glenn shunt. In 1971, Fontan et al. officially published successful cases that treated tricuspid valve atresia through a cavopulmonary connection operation they had been carrying out since 1968 (Fontan and Baudet 1971). Their cavopulmonary connection operation was also known as primitive Fontan surgery. More than 40 years later, a large number of

B. Qiao (✉)
Cardiovascular Institute, General Hospital of Jinan Military Region, Jinan, China

Cardiac Surgery Center, Western District of Shandong Provincial Hospital, Jinan, China

H. J. Li
Institute of Cardiovascular Diseases, Jinan Military Region General Hospital of PLA, Jinan, China

B. Qiao et al. (eds.), *Surgical Atlas of Functional Single Ventricle and Hypoplastic Left Heart Syndrome*, https://doi.org/10.1007/978-981-10-8435-5_7

cardiac surgeons have made improvements and developments to the Fontan connection in different forms. All of these modified methods are collectively referred to as the traditional Fontan procedure, which expands operative indications to other type of functional single ventricle rather than tricuspid valve atresia alone and has become the standard palliation for functional single ventricle surgery. We will introduce these original and modified cavopulmonary connections in this section.

7.2 Cavopulmonary Connection Physiology

The principles of the Fontan procedure used to treat complex cyanotic congenital heart disease are that arterial blood in the systemic circulation and venous blood in pulmonary artery are separated to improve tissue oxygenation, and that the parallel circulation of the single ventricle is switched into a serial circulation by bypassing the right ventricle. Fontan et al. originally used this method to palliate tricuspid valve atresia, and it has subsequently been applied to all types of functional single ventricles and hypoplastic left heart syndrome. As time passed, however, more and more complications of the Fontan connection were notably presented due to disordered blood circulation, including increased vena caval pressure and reduced arterial pressure, as well as systemic venous return obstructions via the cavopulmonary passageway and pulmonary vascular bed. The functional single ventricle could not be filled in diastole, and as a result the ventricular volume load and cardiac output (CO) fell. In order to optimize the physiology of the cavopulmonary connection, Fontan et al. proposed ten operative criteria. They aimed to reduce left atrial and trans-pulmonary artery pressure and to appropriately increase systemic venous pressure in the case that adequate lung flow was maintained.

7.3 Selection Criteria for Fontan Procedure and Risk Factors

To reduce the risk of the cavopulmonary connection, Fontan and his colleagues developed ten strict criteria in 1977 to select patients for Fontan surgery: (1) more than 4 years old; (2) sinus rhythm; (3) normal anatomical systemic veins; (4) normal right atrial volume; (5) pulmonary artery mean pressure lower than 15 mmHg; (6) pulmonary arteriole resistance lower than 4 Wood unit/m^2; (7) more than 0.75 diameter ratio of pulmonary artery to aorta; (8) left ventricular ejection fraction greater than 0.60; (9) normal atrioventricular valve opening and closing; (10) normal pulmonary artery. Over the years, these guidelines have been beneficial to optimize the choice of patients and to increase the success rate of Fontan surgery (Choussat et al. 1978). With the improvement of perioperative care and especially the involvement of hybrid surgery, the criteria were reduced to four items and have been subsequently lowered to one or two items through several rounds of modification.

These changes were initiated in experienced pediatric heart centers. The age restriction was the first change, and now Fontan surgery can be performed before on children younger than 4 years old. Improvement in pacing technology now ensures that non-sinus rhythm is not a contraindication. Right atrial volume is not a restriction because the right atrium can be bypassed. Abnormal systemic venous connections can now be reconstructed or undergo routinely cavopulmonary connections. Pulmonary artery abnormalities can be shaped or revised by stent, and outflow tract stenosis can be corrected by subaortic stenosis resection (or enlargement of the bulboventricular foramen) or application of different sizes of artificial blood vessels. Valve replacement can be performed to deal with atrioventricular valve insufficiency either before or at the same time as the Fontan surgery. As mentioned earlier, the goal of the Fontan circulation physiology is to in principle reduce trans-pulmonary artery pressure, increase acceptable systemic venous pressure, and maintain adequate forward pulmonary blood flow. Therefore, all of the revisions of the criteria for selection of Fontan cases are intended to reduce left atrial pressure and trans-pulmonary artery pressure.

Other problems with Fontan surgery should also be mentioned. The single ventricle can only tolerate mild atrioventricular valve regurgitation. Moderate and severe atrioventricular valve regurgitation will cause the Fontan circulation to fail due to sustaining ventricular volume overload. Another problem is related to the presence of collateral vessels. The collateral circulation can lead to increased pulmonary artery resistance and to changed single ventricular chronic volume load. Fortunately, the formation or replacement of atrioventricular valves and the closure of collateral vessels can be performed by intervention surgery, so these problems can be well resolved.

Notes Classical Glenn shunt surgery ensures that the flow of the superior vena cava returns to right pulmonary circulation, and that mixed blood from the inferior vena cava flows only into left lung circulation. Therefore, this surgery contributes to an elevated oxygen saturation. With a relatively low operative complexity, the procedure does not have to be performed under cardiopulmonary bypass. In olden days, there was a lack of comprehensive understanding of the physiology of the entire cardiovascular system and heart valves. Heart valves at the right atrial inflow and outflow tract play a role in directing blood flow; however, the weak contractility of the right atrium is not enough to keep these two valves closed freely. Additionally, placement of heart valves would extend the time of extracorporeal circulation and valve implantation, and would consequently greatly increase the surgical difficulty, the incidence of complications, and potentially early mortality. So, the development of the original Fontan procedure cannot be continued. In conclusion, the key to a successful treatment of functional single ventricles and to the preservation of persistent palliative effects by Fontan surgery is to quickly predict risks which may result from any possible problems and to reasonably treat them before they occur.

References

Choussat A, Fontan F, Besse F, et al. Selection criteria for Fontan's procedure. In: Anderson R, Shinebourne E, editors. Paediatric cardiology. Edinburgh: Churchill Livingstone; 1978. p. 559–66.

Fontan F, Baudet E. Surgical repair of tricuspid atresia. Thorax. 1971;26(3):240–8. https://doi.org/10.1136/thx.26.3.240.

Haller JA Jr, Adkins JC, Worthington M, Rauenhorst J. Experimental studies on permanent bypass of the right heart. Surgery. 1966;59(6):1128–32. https://doi.org/10.5555/uri:pii:0039606066903217.

Chapter 8
Original Fontan Surgery: One-time Cavopulmonary Connection

Bin Qiao and Feng Quan Zhang

In 1968, Fontan and his colleagues performed the first successful physiological treatment for tricuspid atresia. The mixed blood from the systemic and pulmonary circulations was separated, and the pulmonary blood flow was reconstructed. In 1971, Fontan and his colleagues reported a total of three cases in their publication (Fontan and Baudet 1971). The original Fontan surgery is constituted of five surgical procedures: (1) A classical Glenn shunt, in which the superior vena cava and the right pulmonary artery are divided, followed by an end-to-end anastomosis of the distal end of the superior vena cava to the distal end of the right pulmonary artery; (2) An aortic valve homograft implanted to connect the superior vena caval end of the right atrium and the cardiac end of the right pulmonary artery; (3) The atrial septal defect repaired using a patch; (4) A pulmonary valve homograft implanted in the junction of the inferior vena cava and right atrium; (5) The pulmonary artery trunk is ligated.

Fontan and his colleagues believed that right atrial contraction could drive the blood flow of the inferior vena cava back to the left pulmonary artery, and valves implanted in the inflow and outflow tracts of the right atrium could turn the right atrium into a pump similar to the right ventricle. Their first case belonged to Type Ib tricuspid atresia, with normal relationships between the great arteries, pulmonary hypoplasia, and a small ventricular septal defect (Fig. 8.1).

One of the procedures of the Fontan surgery is a classic Glenn shunt (end-to-end anastomosis between superior vena cava and right pulmonary artery), in which the

B. Qiao (✉)
Cardiovascular Institute, General Hospital of Jinan Military Region, Jinan, China

Cardiac Surgery Center, Western District of Shandong Provincial Hospital, Jinan, China

F. Q. Zhang
Institute of Cardiovascular Diseases, Jinan Military Region General Hospital of PLA, Jinan, China

B. Qiao et al. (eds.), *Surgical Atlas of Functional Single Ventricle and Hypoplastic Left Heart Syndrome*, https://doi.org/10.1007/978-981-10-8435-5_8

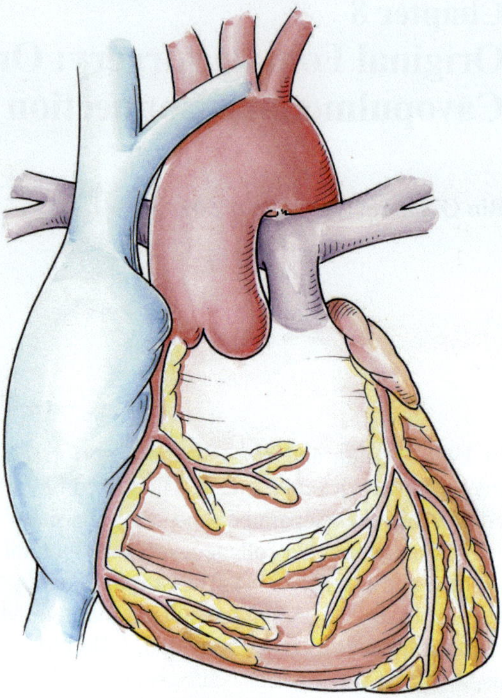

Fig. 8.1 Ib-type tricuspid atresia

distal end of the divided superior vena cava is anastomosed to the distal end of the right pulmonary artery, an allograft valve is implanted in the junction of the inferior vena cava and right atrium, and the pulmonary artery trunk is ligated (Fig. 8.2).

Two more of the cases that Fontan originally reported were also tricuspid atresia, in which the aorta was in front of the left pulmonary artery, and the pulmonary artery was stenotic (Fig. 8.3).

In the two cases previously mentioned, an allogeneic aortic valve was implanted to connect the superior vena caval end of the right atrium and the cardiac end of the right pulmonary artery (Fig. 8.4).

Fontan Circulation Anatomy

The original Fontan procedure connects the right atrium to the pulmonary artery. Fontan et al. believed that the pulse of the right atrium could continuously sustain atrial blood flow to the pulmonary circulation. However, de Leval's experiment showed that, as time went by, the right atrium would expand and gradually lose its systolic function, while eddy currents in the right atrium would result in a decrease in forward pulmonary blood flow via the right atrial pulmonary artery connection. According to de Leval's experimental results, a right atrial pulmonary artery connection was banned in favor of a direct cavopulmonary connection that disregarded the right atrium (de Leval et al. 1988). As a result, systemic venous blood could flow

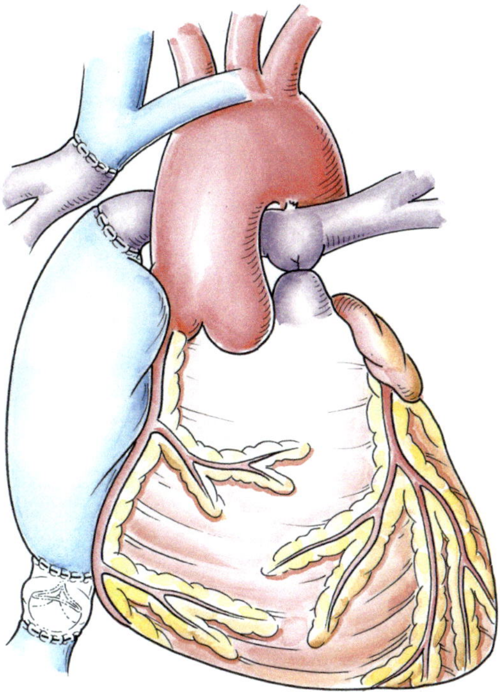

Fig. 8.2 The first case of the original Fontan operation

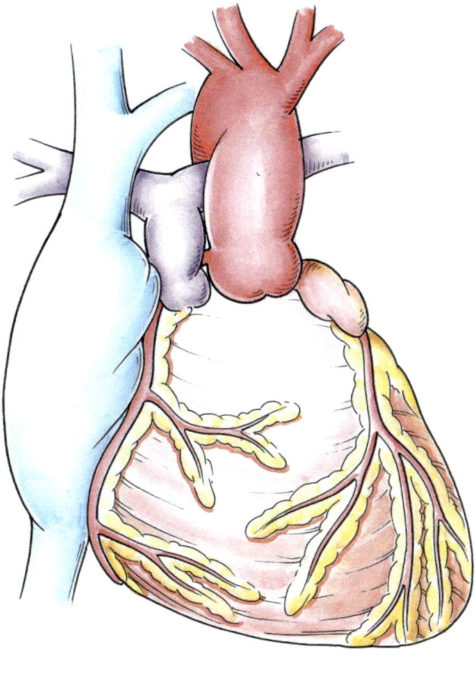

Fig. 8.3 IIIa-type tricuspid atresia

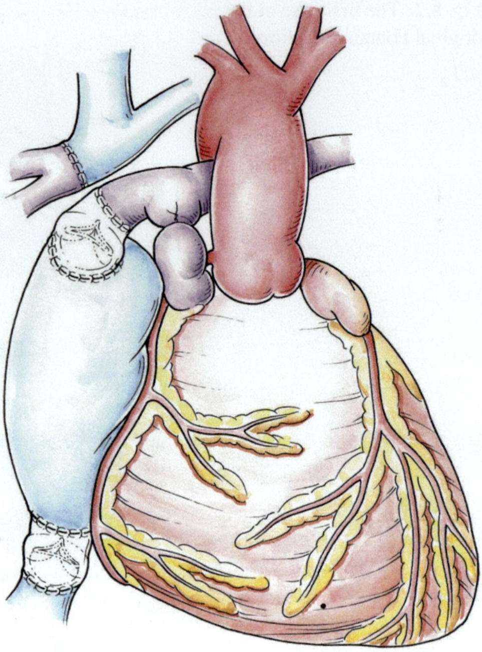

Fig. 8.4 Original Fontan operation: implantation of allogeneic aortic valve

into pulmonary circulation more directly and effectively, and the risk of thrombosis was greatly reduced. This type of circulation with a direct cavopulmonary connection is also known as Fontan circulation. To create the connection, many different methods are used in the clinic, such as conduits with or without valves, homologous grafts, or even direct connections. The materials used for the connection have been modified several times; examples include allogeneic extracardiac conduits with or without valves, other biological tissues, and polytetrafluoroethylene (PTFE).

References

Fontan F, Baudet E. Surgical repair of tricuspid atresia. Thorax. 1971;26(3):240–8. https://doi.org/10.1136/thx.26.3.240.

de Leval MR, Kilner P, Gewillig M, Bull C. Total cavopulmonary connection: A logical alternative to atriopulmonary connection for complex Fontan operations. Experimental studies and early clinical experience. J Thorac Cardiovasc Surg. 1988;96(5):682–95.

Chapter 9
Kreutzer Modified Surgery: Right Atrium Appendage Pulmonary Artery Connection

Bin Qiao, Yan Song Ning, and Zhi Yong Zhang

Kreuzer, who in 1971 was not yet aware of Fontan's creative work, also treated a 3-year-old male patient with tricuspid atresia by performing an anastomosis of the right atrial appendage to the main pulmonary artery. He did not perform a Glenn shunt or use any valves in the inferior vena cava. Additionally, he maintained the size of atrial septal defect to be 6 mm. A Waterston shunt (ascending aorta to right pulmonary artery) performed previously was closed, and thrombosis had been presented in the right pulmonary artery. This was also the first patient to undergo a total pulmonary artery and right atrial connection with fenestration. The operation was named the forward end-to-end right atrial and pulmonary artery connection and was later improved through the use of a homograft with a valve, polyester artificial blood vessels, or an extracardiac conduit without a valve in the connection of the right atrial appendage to the pulmonary artery.

The modified Kreuzer surgery was published in 1973 (Kreutzer et al. 1973).

This figure shows tricuspid atresia with normal aortic positioning. The valve, together with the pulmonary artery main trunk, is anastomosed to the right atrial appendage without performing a Glenn shunt or valvular implantation in the inferior vena cava. A 6mm fenestration is made at the atrial septum. This procedure was called the forward end-to-end connection between right atrium and pulmonary artery (Fig. 9.1).

B. Qiao (✉)
Cardiovascular Institute, General Hospital of Jinan Military Region, Jinan, China

Cardiac Surgery Center, Western District of Shandong Provincial Hospital, Jinan, China

Y. S. Ning
Institute of Cardiovascular Diseases, Jinan Military Region General Hospital of PLA, Jinan, China

Z. Y. Zhang
The 88th Hospital of PLA, Taian, China

B. Qiao et al. (eds.), *Surgical Atlas of Functional Single Ventricle and Hypoplastic Left Heart Syndrome*, https://doi.org/10.1007/978-981-10-8435-5_9

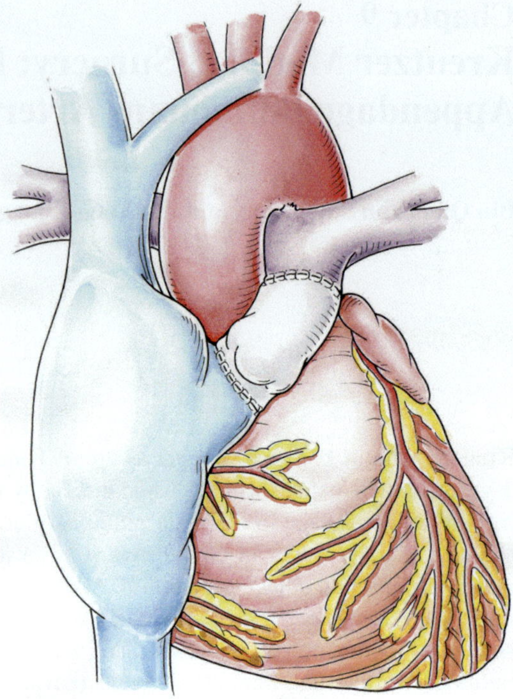

Fig. 9.1 Kreutzer modified surgery: the connection between right atrium appendage and pulmonary artery by conduit with valve

In the improved method, a polyester extracardiac conduit was used to connect the pulmonary artery to the right atrial appendage (Fig. 9.2).

For cases with transposition of the great arteries in which the pulmonary artery is on the right side of the aorta, it is relatively simple to connect the pulmonary artery to the right atrial appendage. Surgery is performed under cardiopulmonary bypass at room temperature without blocking the ascending aorta and under beating-heart conditions. The left and right pulmonary arteries are blocked immediately after commencing cardiopulmonary bypass. The operation is further simplified if there is not a pulmonary valve. The pulmonary artery close to the pulmonary valve is divided, followed by tightening of the superior and inferior vena cava cannulas. After division, the right atrial appendage is anastomosed to the pulmonary artery. Continuous suturing is used, starting from the rear wall. Continuous 6-0 Prolene is preferable in children. The proximal end of the pulmonary artery is oversewn with continuous suturing (Fig. 9.3).

The Figure 9.4 shows the end-to-end connection between the pulmonary artery and right atrial appendage at the conclusion of the operation, without the implantation of valves in either the connection or the inferior vena cava.

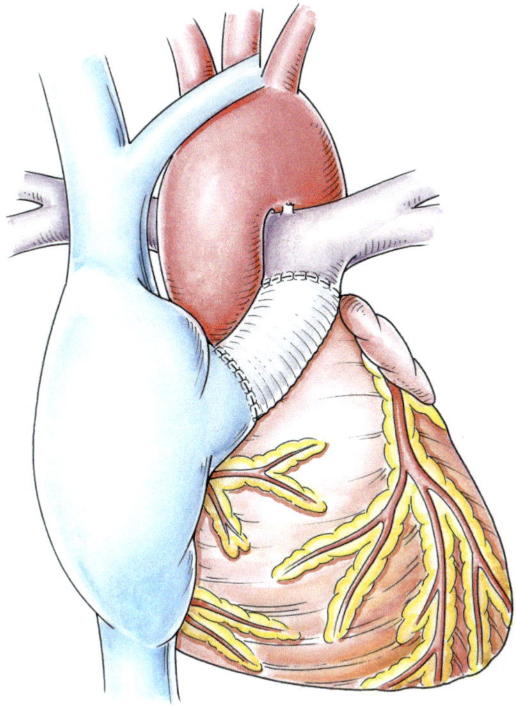

Fig. 9.2 Kreutzer modified surgery: the connection between right atrium appendage and pulmonary artery by polyester extracardiac conduit

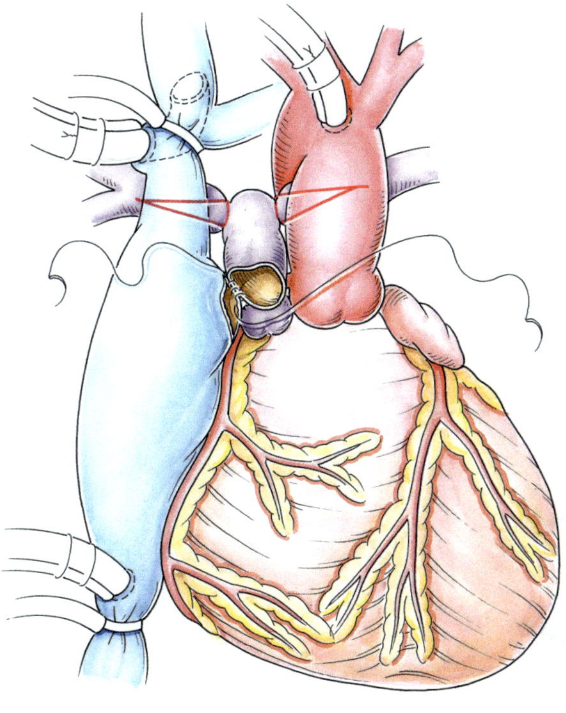

Fig. 9.3 Kreutzer modified surgery: end-end anastomosis of right atrium appendage and pulmonary artery

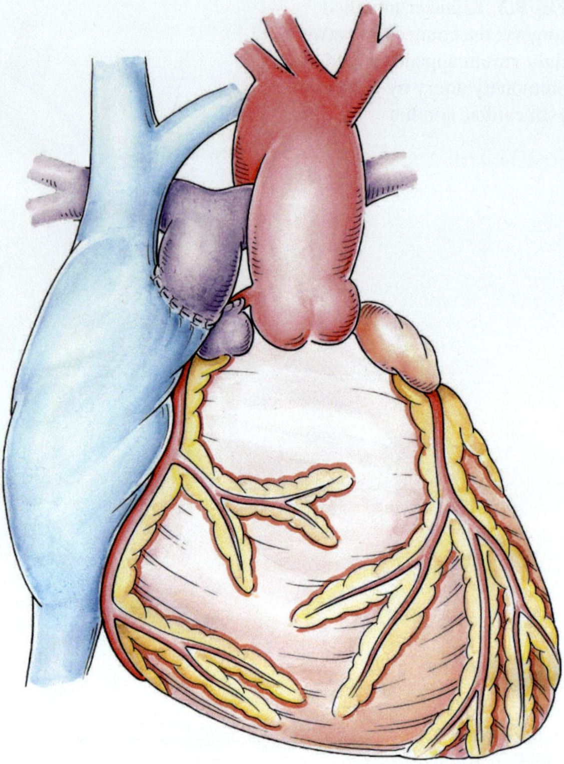

Fig. 9.4 Kreutzer modified surgery: end-end anastomosis completed

Reference

Kreutzer G, Galíndez E, Bono H, De PC, Laura JP. An operation for the correction of tricuspid atresia. J Thorac Cardiovasc Surg. 1973;66(4):613–21.

Chapter 10
Björk Modified Surgery: Right Atrium Right Ventricle Connection

Bin Qiao, Wen Yuan Duan, and Yi Fei Hua

During a period of ten years after the commencement of Fontan's and Kreuzer's operations, the original Fontan surgery and Kreuzer's modified surgery were widely used to treat tricuspid valve atresia. In 1978, concerning the forward end-to-end connection between the right atrial appendage and pulmonary artery, a new surgical method of a backward connection of the right atrium to the pulmonary artery was proposed in order to minimize compression of the sternum on the pulmonary artery due to the fact that some of these arteries are located behind the ascending aorta. This new surgical method was soon accepted. However, pulmonary valval calcification, degeneration, and stenosis had a negative impact on blood flow in the pulmonary artery and right atrial connection, so the valve was generally not implanted. At that time, because patients were selected to undergo the original Fontan surgery in accordance with Fontan's 10 criteria, many children more than 4 years old were in very bad condition when undergoing surgery, and the failure rate of the operation was very high. Therefore, some surgeons conceived the idea of bringing the infant right ventricle into the pulmonary circulation. They believed that the basic systolic function of the right ventricle was available, even if it was very weak. In 1978, Bowman et al. employed an extracardiac conduit with heterotopic swine heart valves in a connection between the right atrium and the right ventricle to establish forward blood flow and found that the volume of the right ventricular cavity

B. Qiao (✉)
Cardiovascular Institute, General Hospital of Jinan Military Region, Jinan, China

Cardiac Surgery Center, Western District of Shandong Provincial Hospital, Jinan, China

W. Y. Duan
Institute of Cardiovascular Diseases, Jinan Military Region General Hospital of PLA, Jinan, China

Y. F. Hua
Shanghai Dongfang Hospital, Tongji University, Shanghai, China

B. Qiao et al. (eds.), *Surgical Atlas of Functional Single Ventricle and Hypoplastic Left Heart Syndrome*, https://doi.org/10.1007/978-981-10-8435-5_10

increased (Bowman et al. 1978). Other surgeons quickly and successfully replicated this surgical method, incorporating with it repair of atrial and ventricular septal defects and relief of pulmonary artery stenosis in order to implement an entire tricuspid valve atresia repair. However, while the homograft or xenograft extracardiac valved conduit had the inherent disadvantages described above, it could also not tolerate the growth of children. In 1979, Björk et al. modified the surgery further. The right atrial appendage, alongside a part of the right atrial posterior wall, was anastomosed to the opening of the right ventricle to form the posterior wall of a right atrial-right ventricular channel, while the anterior wall of the channel was formed used autologous pericardium (Björk et al. 1979). Some surgeries continued to implant valves in right atrial-right ventricular channel in the Björk modified operation. However, the Björk modified operation could not be further promoted due to the possibility of the sternum compressing the right atrial-right ventricular outflow tract after chest had been closed.

It is suitable for most patients who suffer from tricuspid atresia without pulmonary stenosis to undergo Björk modified surgery. The surgery should be carried out under cardiopulmonary bypass. Cardioplegia, blockage of the ascending aorta, and cardiac arrest are necessary with respect to the closure of the atrial septal defect and ventricular septal defect. The right ventricle is longitudinally incised under the pulmonary valve while avoiding injury of the coronary arteries across the ventricular surface. The ventricular septal defect can generally be closed through the incision. The three sides of the right atrium are incised and opened to form an auricular flap near the right atrial appendage. The posterior wall of the channel from the right atrium to the right ventricle is constructed by suturing the free edge of the atrial wall flap with the adjacent edge of the ventricular incision using a continuous suture. Because the incision in the right atrium is large, the atrial septal defect can be closed through it using a patch (Fig. 10.1).

After the previous step, the right atrium and the right ventricle are open. The right atrial-right ventricular outflow tract is completed by covering the top surface of the atrial wall flap using autologous pericardium. The channel is shaped like a half pipe when completed. An autologous pericardial patch was used by Björk during the development of the procedure, although other materials such as Gore-Tex patches are used by some surgeons (Fig. 10.2).

In Björk's improved surgery, the cavopulmonary connection is composed of a part of the atrial appendage wall, as well as some pericardial patch. In light of the special design of the right atrial and right ventricular incisions, it can be difficult to suture the channel. In particular, the rear wall of the channel consists of atrium, atrial appendage, and right ventricular wall, but they are inconsistent in thickness and do not lie in a straight line. Therefore, they are not likely to be tightly connected with the pericardium. Blood leakage is often present, and it is difficult and time consuming to repair. Some surgeons use valved or non-valved conduits

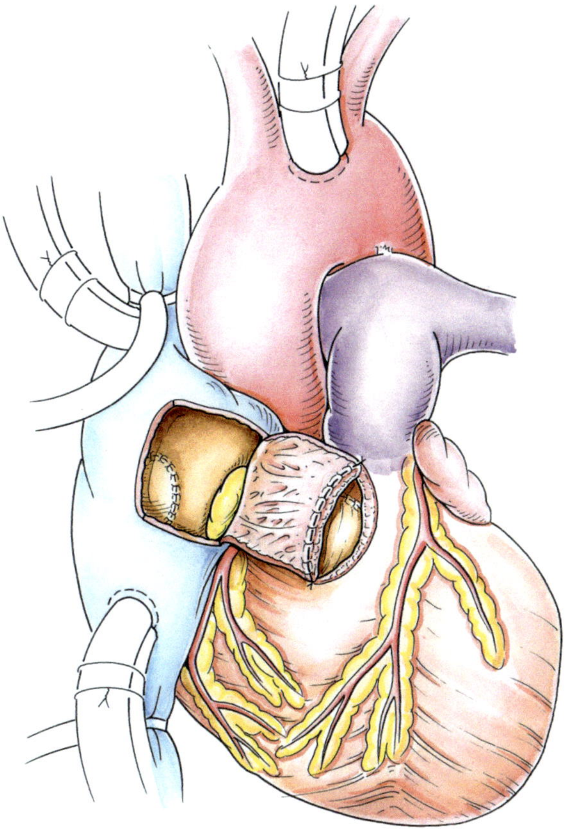

Fig. 10.1 Björk modified surgery: posterior wall of right atrial-right ventricular channel

directly to connect the right atrium and right ventricle by making parallel incisions on the anterior walls of the right atrial appendage and right ventricle. The incision diameter should correspond with the connecting conduit and should be at least more than double the diameter of the vena cava. Closure of the atrial septal and ventricular septal defects can be performed through these two incisions (Fig. 10.3).

Only the diameter of the conduit needs to be considered when using a non-valved external conduit. When using a valved external conduit, however, the conduit diameter and valve size, as well as the valve opening direction, should be confirmed before suturing. The valve should be placed in the middle of conduit. If positioned too close to the atrial or ventricular opening, the valve's shape can deform when anastomosing and subsequently increase resistance to blood flow and reduce the durability of the valve (Fig. 10.4).

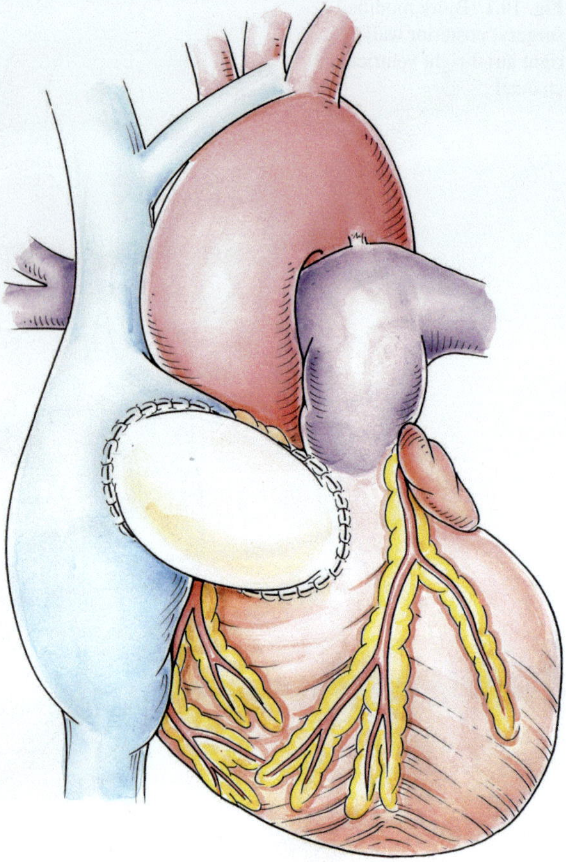

Fig. 10.2 Björk modified surgery: anterior wall of right atrial-right ventricular channel

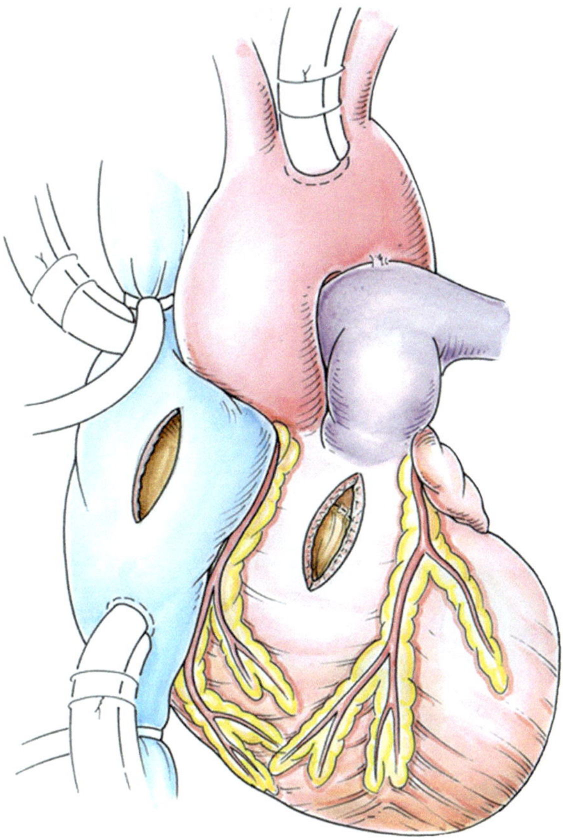

Fig. 10.3 Björk modified surgery: right atrium and right ventricular incision

Fig. 10.4 Björk modified surgery: connecting right atrium and right ventricle by conduit with flap

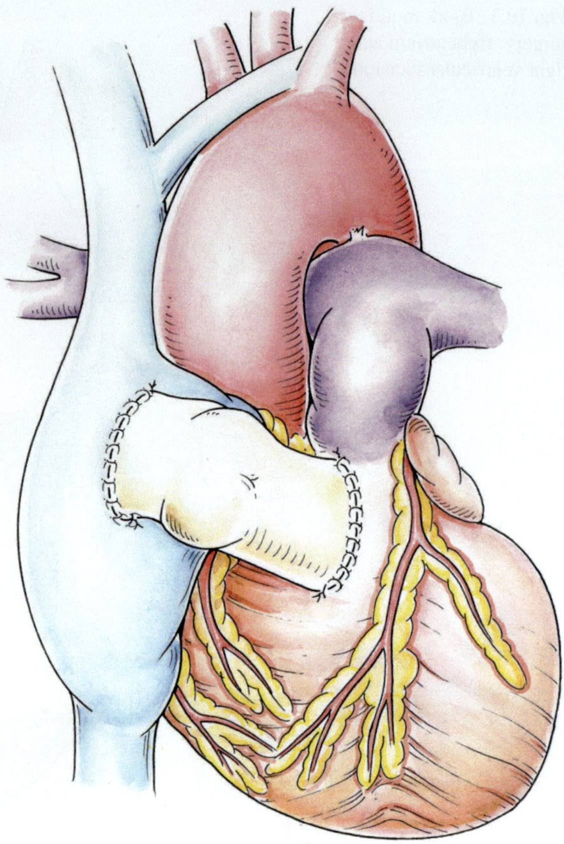

References

Björk VO, Olin CL, Bjarke BB, Thorén CA. Right atrial-right ventricular anastomosis for correction of tricuspid atresia. J Thorac Cardiovasc Surg. 1979;77(3):452–8.

Bowman FO, Malm JR, Hayes CJ, Gersony WM. Physiological approach to surgery for tricuspid atresia. Circulation. 1978;58(3 Pt 2):I83–6.

Chapter 11
Norwood Modified Surgery: Right Atrium Pulmonary Artery Connection

Bin Qiao and Shi Feng Liu

The modified Norwood surgery must be performed under cardiopulmonary bypass. The cannulas should be placed in the junction of the superior vena cava and innominate vein. Intubation of the inferior vena cava should be near the diaphragm. Because of the presence of an atrial septal defect, cardioplegia should be employed. Ventricular fibrillation is induced following blockage of the ascending aorta or under cardiopulmonary bypass. The right pulmonary artery can be exposed by pulling the ascending aorta and superior vena cava away. A 2 cm (depending on right pulmonary artery size) incision is made along the right pulmonary artery in the midline of its anterior wall. A curved incision is made along the anterior wall of the superior vena cava, extending to the right atrium away from the sinoatrial node, which is present at the junction of right atrium and superior vena cava. The last step is to cut the main pulmonary artery to open, find the pulmonary valve, and close the valve by suture (Fig. 11.1).

The atrial septal defect, which can be exposed through the incision of the right atrium, is closed with a suitable patch. The continuous suture is tightened at the rear wall of the pulmonary artery and right atrial connection, and knots are tied at both ends. After the pulmonary valve is closed, the incision at the main trunk of the pulmonary artery is closed by continuous suture (Fig. 11.2).

The incision of the pulmonary artery and right atrium remains open. A part of the pulmonary artery and the right atrium is selected as the rear wall of the connection port between the pulmonary artery and right atrium. To facilitate suturing, the right

B. Qiao (✉)
Cardiovascular Institute, General Hospital of Jinan Military Region, Jinan, China

Cardiac Surgery Center, Western District of Shandong Provincial Hospital, Jinan, China

S. F. Liu
Institute of Cardiovascular Diseases, Jinan Military Region General Hospital of PLA, Jinan, China

B. Qiao et al. (eds.), *Surgical Atlas of Functional Single Ventricle and Hypoplastic Left Heart Syndrome*, https://doi.org/10.1007/978-981-10-8435-5_11

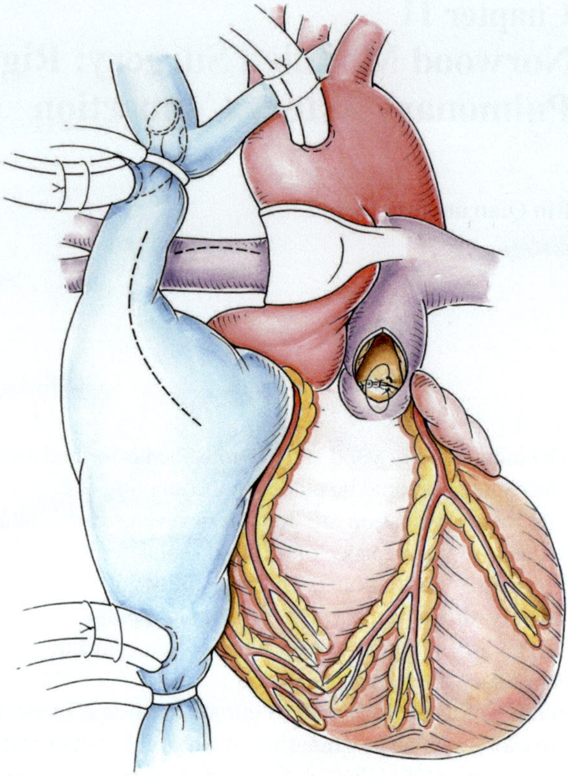

Fig. 11.1 Norwood modified surgery: incision on pulmonary artery, incision from anterior wall of superior vena cava to right atrium, suturing pulmonary valve

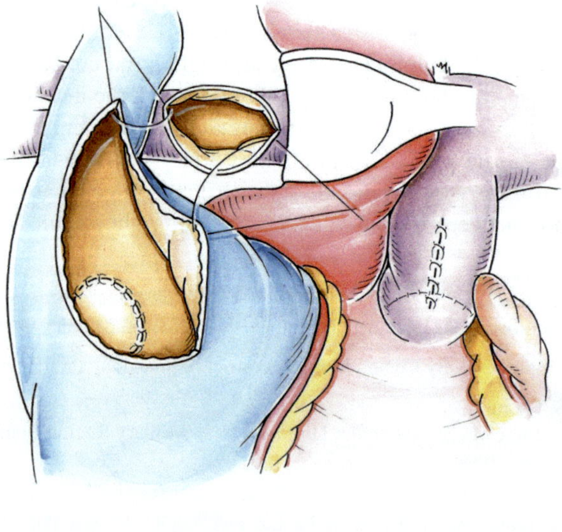

Fig. 11.2 Norwood modified surgery: atrium septum closed, anastomosing right atrium and pulmonary artery

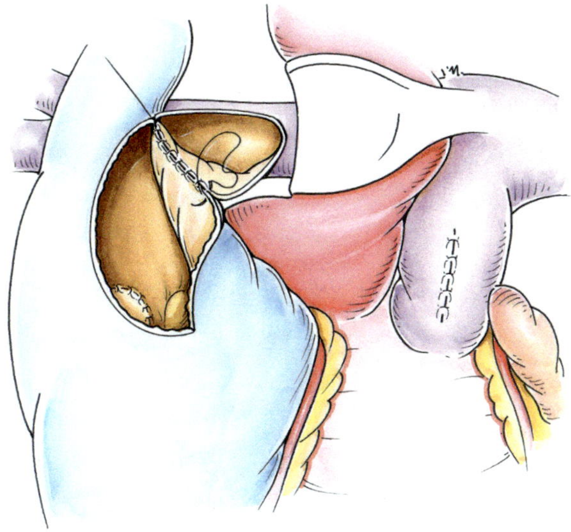

Fig. 11.3 Norwood modified surgery: right atrium and pulmonary artery anastomosis completed

atrial wall is selected according to the size of the pulmonary artery incision, sutures are pre-set at the corresponding parts, and knots are tied. Continuous suturing is performed to complete the rear wall. Note that the connection port is at least 50% greater than vena cava in diameter in order to ensure that blood return from the superior vena cava and inferior vena cava is unobstructed in later Fontan operations (Fig. 11.3).

The uncompleted anastomosis of the atrium and pulmonary artery is anteriorly covered with a patch of Gore-Tex material. After venting air, we can reopen the superior and inferior venae cavae (Fig. 11.4).

Notes The total cavopulmonary connection is idealized in the Norwood modified operation; however, it is different than the modified Björk operation in which the conduit directly in front of the heart would be compressed when closing the chest.

The modified Norwood total cavopulmonary connection has also been used in the treatment of hypoplastic left heart syndrome. At that time, surgical treatment for either functional single ventricle or hypoplastic left heart syndrome was a one-step process. Because of the degradation of the myocardium and the decrease of ventricular diastolic volume after palliation, the early mortality rate was high, and the long-term survival rate was low. Having understood these pathological changes, physicians have gradually adopted the staged surgery. Norwood, before completing the connection of the right atrium to the pulmonary artery, pre-set a patch in the superior vena caval inlet in the atrium to isolate the inferior vena caval blood to the pulmonary artery, allowing only the superior vena caval blood to flow into the pulmonary artery. To accomplish this, the atrial septal defect should be kept large

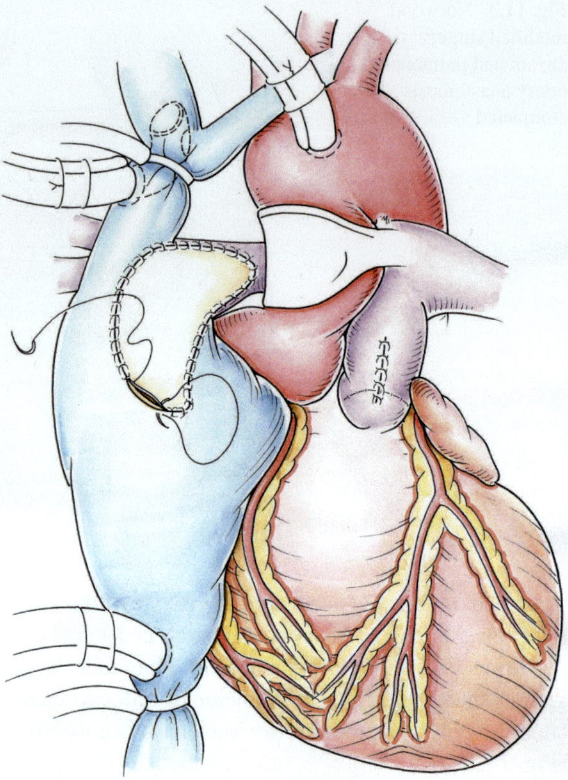

Fig. 11.4 Norwood modified surgery: patching anastomotic anterior wall of right atrium and pulmonary artery

enough to allow blood from the inferior vena cava to pass through it into bodily circulation. The modified Norwood operation has also been called the hemi-Fontan surgery, considering the fact that it would become a real cavopulmonary connection after the patch had been removed and the atrial septal defect had been closed. It is also known as Norwood II surgery in the treatment of hypoplastic left heart syndrome. The hemi-Fontan surgery designed for the treatment of functional single ventricle and hemi-Fontan surgery designed for hypoplastic left heart syndrome, i.e., Norwood II surgery, will be described in Chaps. 14 and 26.

Chapter 12
de Leval Modified Surgery

Bin Qiao and Bao Wei Shao

In 1988, after a wide range of studies on loss of function after the enlargement of the right atrium in atriopulmonary anastomoses, de Leval proposed the concept of an intra-atrial lateral tunnel Fontan circulation (de Leval et al. 1988). They separated all or most of the right atrium and right ventricle from the Fontan circulation. The surgery consisted of three procedures: (1) two end-to-side anastomoses, i.e., the divided superior vena cava to the superior and inferior surfaces of the right pulmonary artery, by bypassing the right atrium and the right ventricle; (2) an intracardiac tunnel was constructed using the posterolateral wall of the right atrium; (3) along the posterior wall of atrium, a semi-pipe patch was sutured from the inferior vena cava to the anastomosis between the proximal end of the superior vena cava and the right pulmonary artery. Its advantages are enumerated as follows: (1) The operation was simple, without requiring the consideration of the type of anatomical connection. (2) The bypassing of right atrium could prevent atrial dilation because of the high venous pressure. (3) The resulting linear blood flow could reduce the energy consumption of the heart, turbulent flow, and consequent risk of atrial thrombosis. In addition, balanced distribution of blood flow to left and right lungs could be obtained. (4) Compared with an extracardiac conduit cavopulmonary connection, the intra-atrial tunnel maintained the growth potential of the atrium and vena cava in small patients. (5) All of the pressure gradients across the cavopulmonary anastomoses were at a minimum. This was the earliest total cavopulmonary surgery. The intra-atrial

B. Qiao (✉)
Cardiovascular Institute, General Hospital of Jinan Military Region, Jinan, China

Cardiac Surgery Center, Western District of Shandong Provincial Hospital, Jinan, China

B. W. Shao
Institute of Cardiovascular Diseases, Jinan Military Region General Hospital of PLA, Jinan, China

B. Qiao et al. (eds.), *Surgical Atlas of Functional Single Ventricle and Hypoplastic Left Heart Syndrome*, https://doi.org/10.1007/978-981-10-8435-5_12

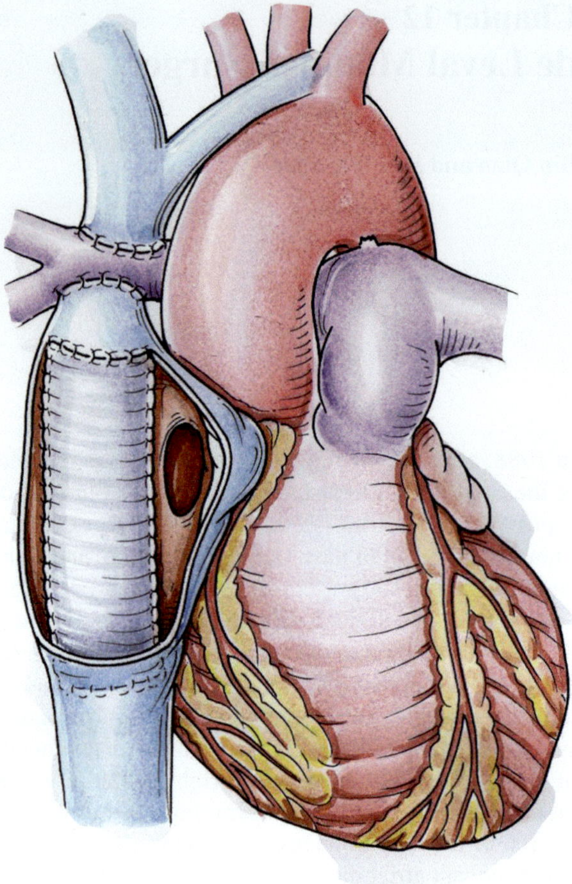

Fig. 12.1 de Leval improved surgery: intra-atrial lateral tunnel cavopulmonary connection

tunnel could also be replaced by an intra-atrial conduit which directly connected the inferior vena cava to the pulmonary trunk. The twenty cases who underwent the de Leval modified operation were diagnosed as follows: double inlet ventricle, right heart dysplasia, and tricuspid valve atresia. Potential risks still presented in the de Leval modified Fontan connection, such as atrial dilatation and postoperative atrial arrhythmias. These complications could be related to the suturing technique of the intra-atrial tunnel. The operative procedure required extracorporeal bypass, cardioplegia, blockage of the ascending aorta, and cardiac arrest.

The original de Leval modified Fontan surgery required extracorporeal bypass, cardioplegia, blockage of the ascending aorta, and cardiac arrest. The whole procedure includes: (1) two end-to-side anastomoses, i.e., the divided superior vena cava to the superior and inferior surfaces of the right pulmonary artery, by bypassing right atrium and right ventricle; (2) an intracardiac tunnel constructed using the posterolateral wall of the right atrium; (3) along the posterior wall of atrium, a semi-

Fig. 12.2 de Leval improved surgery: intra-atrial conduit cavopulmonary connection

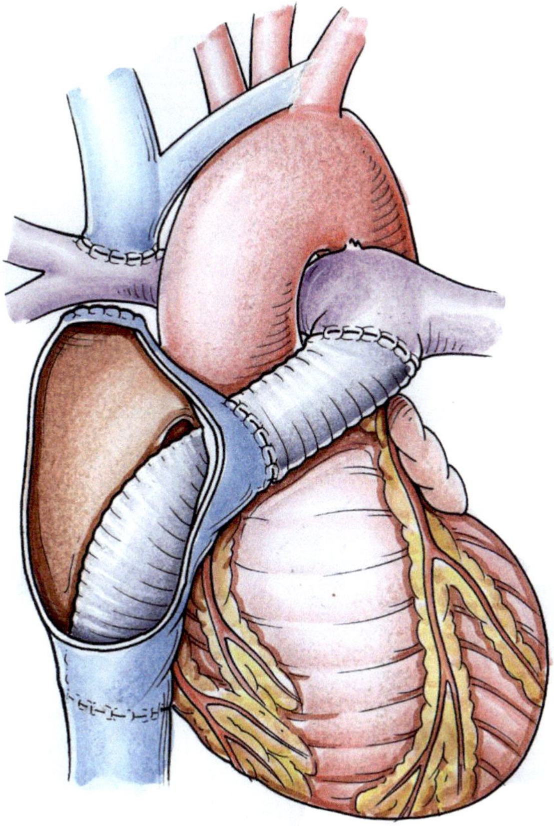

pipe patch sutured from the inferior vena cava to the anastomosis of the proximal end of the superior vena cava to the right pulmonary artery; (4) if the atrial septal defect is not large, it should be enlarged (Fig. 12.1).

The intra-atrial lateral tunnel total cavopulmonary connection can also be replaced by an intra-atrial artificial conduit connection. The procedure is described as follows. The superior vena cava is divided, and its distal end is anastomosed to the right pulmonary artery, while its cardiac end is continuously oversewn. If the atrial septal defect is too small, it should be enlarged following the opening of the right atrium. The artificial conduit should be suited for the inferior vena cava and its anastomosis. After exiting the right atrial appendage, the conduit is anastomosed to the pulmonary artery (Fig. 12.2).

Notes The modern intra-atrial tunnel Fontan procedure has actually evolved from the de Leval operation. Another contribution made by de Leval showed that collisions between the superior and inferior vena cava in the atrium can cause flow turbulence in the atriopulmonary connection, which can be further intensified by the beating of the heart. The intra-atrial total cavopulmonary connection proposed by de

Leval is superior to the right atrial pulmonary artery connection, as well as to many other connections. In addition, he proposed the possibility of an extracardiac conduit total cavopulmonary connection.

Reference

de Leval MR, Kilner P, Gewillig M, Bull C. Total cavopulmonary connection: A logical alternative to atriopulmonary connection for complex Fontan operations. Experimental studies and early clinical experience. J Thorac Cardiovasc Surg. 1988;96(5):682–95.

Chapter 13
Staged Fontan Surgery

Bin Qiao and Yan Song Ning

Over the past two decades, more and more modifications to the Fontan surgery brightened the treatment of functional single ventricle, and reports on successful palliation were continuously published. However, the early surgical mortality rate was still high, and postoperative complications were difficult to treat, even if a restricted selection of patients had been made according to the Fontan criteria. These complications included: increased central venous pressure, arrhythmia, pleural effusion, ascites, edema, etc. Supplementation of volume to elevate low arterial blood pressure would increase venous pressure; in turn, the application of vasodilators would further lower arterial pressure, and eventually patients would die of heart failure. From echocardiographic follow-up results, it was observed that the ventricular wall gradually thickened, and that ventricular volume gradually lessened over time regardless of heart function. These results implied that the blood circulation of the functional single ventricle had been converted into Fontan circulation after palliation, characterized by the chronic pre-surgical ascension of ventricular volume suddenly decreasing after surgery, the rapid degeneration of myocardial quality, and the subsequent decrease of ventricular diastolic volume. In view of this pathophysiologic change, pediatric cardiologists proposed a staged procedure in place of the original one-step total cavopulmonary Fontan procedure in an effort to reduce or even avoid myocardial quality degradation and ventricular diastolic volume decrease after palliative surgery.

B. Qiao (✉)
Cardiovascular Institute, General Hospital of Jinan Military Region, Jinan, China

Cardiac Surgery Center, Western District of Shandong Provincial Hospital, Jinan, China

Y. S. Ning
Institute of Cardiovascular Diseases, Jinan Military Region General Hospital of PLA, Jinan, China

B. Qiao et al. (eds.), *Surgical Atlas of Functional Single Ventricle and Hypoplastic Left Heart Syndrome*, https://doi.org/10.1007/978-981-10-8435-5_13

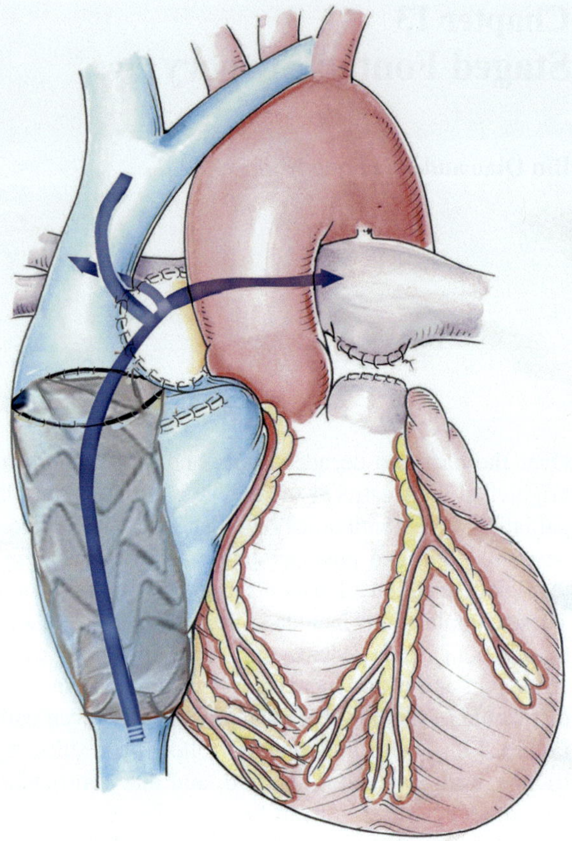

Fig. 13.1 Blood flow direction after stage II Fontan surgery by intervention method

Various staged Fontan operations had been carried out by many cardiac surgeons using different methods in the late 1980s and early 1990s. In principle, by the first stage of palliation, the superior vena caval blood was conducted to the pulmonary artery, while the inferior vena caval blood mixed with a part of the oxygenated arterial blood and also traveled to the pulmonary artery; by the second stage of palliation, the direct connection between the inferior vena cava and pulmonary artery was performed. The staged procedures can be summarized as follows:

1. The bidirectional Glenn shunt provides a better surgical option for patients who cannot take original Fontan surgery because of high-risk factors. For these patients, the bidirectional Glenn can be performed as an intermediate palliation to reduce complications and mortality rates of the Fontan surgery. Additionally, with the Glenn shunt, the Fontan operation can be conducted as early as 4 years old. After the completion of a bidirectional Glenn shunt, most surgeons selectively adopted an extracardiac conduit to connect the inferior vena cava with the pulmonary artery, and to bypass the right atrium.

2. In 1989, Norwood believed that since the total cavopulmonary connection would be eventually completed, a passage connecting the right atrium and the pulmonary artery (i.e., early right atrial pulmonary artery connection) was constructed in advance, followed by a blockage of inferior vena caval blood while allowing superior vena caval blood to pass through the passage into the pulmonary artery. In the second stage, the so-called intra-atrial conduit Fontan procedure was performed solely by removing the barrier which blocked the inferior vena caval flow from the pulmonary artery and by separating the right atrium with a patch (Norwood 1991). The operation designed by Norwood is actually an intermediate stage of the Fontan procedure, so it is also called the hemi-Fontan procedure; a total cavopulmonary connection is collectively referred to as the full Fontan procedure.

Following the hemi-Fontan operation, the stage II Fontan operation is often performed through a surgical procedure. Surgeons attempted to open the patch previously separating the inferior vena cava. Then, they implanted a large vascular artificial stent which not only connects inferior vena cava to pulmonary artery but also separates the left and right atrium. Of note, the separating patch adopted in the hemi-Fontan operation should be made of biological materials which can be punctured and should have a metal ring around it to facilitate the fixation of the large vascular stent in the interventional process. The above figure illustrates the blood flow direction of the total cavopulmonary connection. In fact, many doctors have directly attempted to implant the stent by an interventional technique after hemi-Fontan surgery, so it is necessary to design a cut of the patch through which blood from the inferior vena cava can flow into the pulmonary artery, as well as the subsequent implantation method of the stent in hemi-Fontan surgery.

Reference

Norwood WI. Hypoplastic left heart syndrome. Ann Thorac Surg. 1991;52(3):688–95.

Chapter 14
Hemi-Fontan Surgery and Intra-atrial Lateral Tunnel Fontan Surgery: Staged Right Atrium Pulmonary Artery Connection

Bin Qiao and Jian Shi Liu

The hemi-Fontan operation is another option, like the bidirectional Glenn shunt, of choice to be an intermediate operation to complete the ultimate total cavopulmonary Fontan connection with an intra-atrial lateral tunnel. It is more appropriate for patients with pulmonary artery insufficiency or stenosis.

Because sick children are mostly dysplasic and weigh less than normal children, the hemi-Fontan operation is performed at the level of the atrium and pulmonary artery. Because the patients with single ventricular defects frequently have rich collateral circulation in the lung, a large amount of pulmonary backflow would affect surgical procedures under routine cardiopulmonary bypass, so the hemi-Fontan surgery is better carried out under deep hypothermic and circulatory arrest. A median sternotomy incision is the most generally used approach. The ascending aorta is conventionally intubated. Single intubation is placed at the right atrial appendage for vena cava intubation. It can be removed during circulatory arrest and re-inserted when cardiopulmonary bypass is ready to be restored. Intravenous intubations can also be placed in the superior and inferior venae cavae, as far toward their distal ends as possible, which should not affect the operation during either circulatory arrest or parallel circulation. The aortopulmonary shunt should be dissected before extracorporeal circulation and be closed immediately after the start of extracorporeal circulation to avoid lung perfusion. Cycle stoppage time should last up to 60 min under deep hypothermia conditions with an anal and rectal temperature of 16–18 °C. The period between extracorporeal circulation and deep hypothermia is recommended to be at least 20 min. When the cycle has stopped, the whole-body blood should be retrieved

B. Qiao (✉)
Cardiovascular Institute, General Hospital of Jinan Military Region, Jinan, China

Cardiac surgery center, Western District of Shandong Provincial Hospital, Jinan, China

J. S. Liu
Tianjin Thoracic Hospital, Tianjin, China

B. Qiao et al. (eds.), *Surgical Atlas of Functional Single Ventricle and Hypoplastic Left Heart Syndrome*, https://doi.org/10.1007/978-981-10-8435-5_14

in an extracorporeal circulation machine. With temperature decreasing, the heart will naturally stop beating. To effectively protect the myocardium, cardioplegia is applied according to the surgeon's own experience after the ascending aorta has been blocked. Experienced pediatric cardiac surgeons tend to apply hypothermic cardiopulmonary bypass with an anal and rectal temperature of around 22 °C, with the superior and inferior venae cavae intubated. The arterial infusion of extracorporeal circulation can be one-third of normal perfusion volume. The bypass can be temporarily stopped for a few minutes when the lung blood is too much and continued after the relative procedure has been completed. Whether using moderate or deep hypothermia bypass, systemic blood vessels immediately constrict once cooling begins; resistance increases accordingly, and cooling time is subsequently prolonged. Generally, vasodilators should be intravenously administered before cardiopulmonary bypass so that the systemic vasculature will dilate to improve the cooling rate.

The hemi-Fontan surgery was initially designed by Norwood for hypoplastic left heart syndrome. In the first stage of the cavopulmonary anastomosis, the pulmonary artery only accepts blood flow from the systemic vein. The pulmonary artery can be divided into functional single ventricle, especially when accompanied with pulmonary stenosis or hypoplasia. With regard to the intracardiac operation, the hemi-Fontan procedure should be carried out under cardiopulmonary bypass, conventional intubation of the aorta and inferior and superior venae cavae, moderate hypothermia, and cardiac arrest. Figure 14.1 shows a small pulmonary trunk and pulmonary stenosis. A transverse incision on the main trunk of the pulmonary artery is also marked. The right atrial incision starts from the upper front of the appendage, circumvents the coronary sinus, advances upward along the medial side of the superior vena cava, and ends approximately 3–4 mm above the pulmonary artery incision. The right pulmonary artery incision is made in the front of right pulmonary artery; its right end is close to the superior vena cava and extends along the vessel to a site just under the ascending aorta, or to the junction of the left and right pulmonary arteries if the right pulmonary artery is small. The incision of the right pulmonary artery is almost perpendicular to the incision at the superior vena cava and right atrium.

The right side of the pulmonary incision is anastomosed to the superior vena cava using 6-0 continuous Prolene, beginning from the middle of the anastomosis, upward to the top of the superior vena cava, and downward to the atrial entrance of the superior vena cava (Fig. 14.2).

The patch of autologous pericardial or pulmonary artery allogeneic graft is shaped like a diamond. This patch acts not only as the front wall of the anastomosis, but also as a separation between the superior vena cava and inferior vena cava. The anastomosis of the inferior edge of the right pulmonary artery incision to the patch is performed from the left end of the right pulmonary artery incision to the lowest point of the cavopulmonary suture that has previously been made. The patch suturing is continued at the same level, extending along the edge of the atrial entrance of

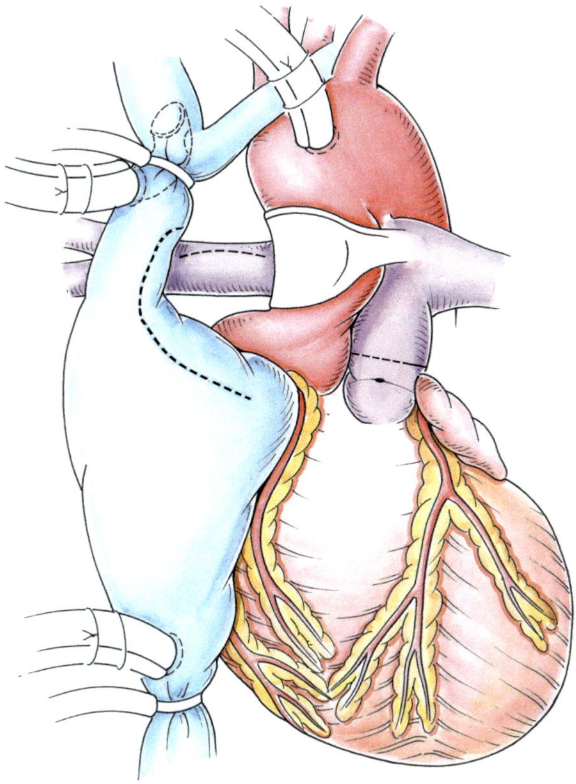

Fig. 14.1 Hemi-Fontan surgery: the incision of pulmonary trunk, right atrium, and right pulmonary artery

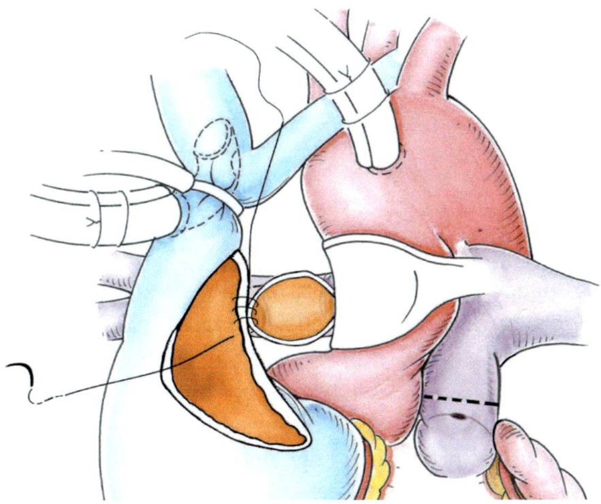

Fig. 14.2 Hemi-Fontan surgery: the anastomosis of right atrium with pulmonary artery

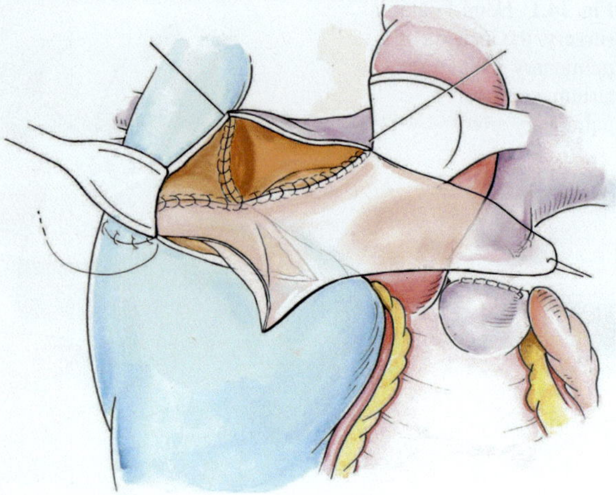

Fig. 14.3 Hemi-Fontan surgery: patch suture 1

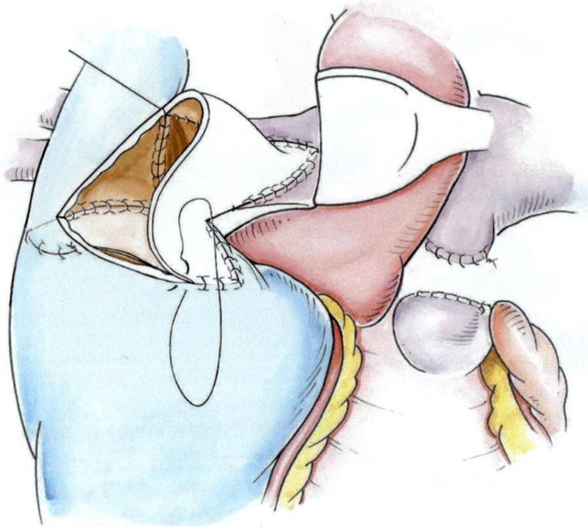

Fig. 14.4 Hemi-Fontan surgery: patch suture 2

the superior vena cava to the middle of the right atrial incision, also using continuous 6-0 Prolene. Finish by tightening with knots (Fig. 14.3).

The patch is now flipped over. This procedure is intended to continue suturing the superior edge of the patch with the superior edge of the right pulmonary artery incision using the first needle of the suture which has been left at its left end. The patch is then lifted up. Its free edge is folded at a 90° angle to itself, and suturing is continued at the left lower edge of the right atrial incision to its lower end with another suture. The two-folded layer of the patch and the right atrial incision wall are sutured together. By folding the patch, communication between the superior vena cava and right atrium is closed (Fig. 14.4). It is then time to begin cardiopulmonary bypass

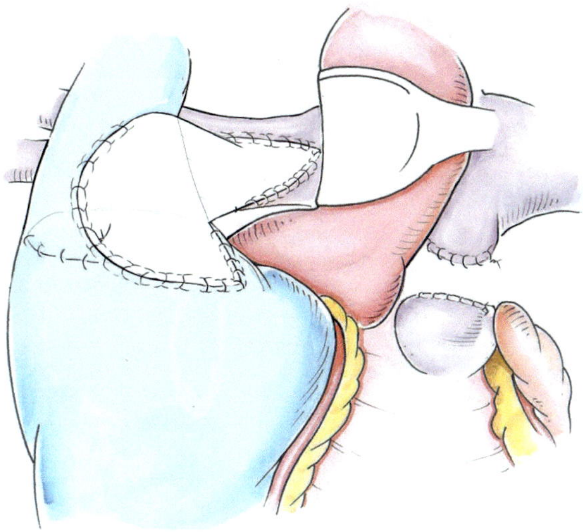

Fig. 14.5 Hemi-Fontan surgery: surgery completed

and gradual warming if in deep hypothermic and circulatory arrest. The suturing of the patch can finally be completed during the rewarming period, which normally lasts 45 min. If moderate hypothermia bypass has been used, flow can be increased to normal levels, rewarming the body. Generally, heart beating will automatically gradually restore from a slow heart rate (HR) to a normal one when the myocardial temperature reaches 24–26 °C. If heart beating remains slow and weak, it may be appropriate to drip ten times diluted epinephrine on the surface of the heart. Cardiopulmonary bypass is considered to end when anal and rectal temperature has reached 37 °C. The protocol to operate cardiopulmonary bypass could follow the one for regular open-heart surgery. In general, the heart function is capable of driving the systemic circulation. However, it is worth noticing that oxygen saturation has to be monitored and kept above 80%.

After the completion of the patch suturing, the patch becomes the front wall of the cavopulmonary anastomosis in hemi-Fontan surgery. This surgery is designed to facilitate eventual intracardiac lateral tunnel total Fontan surgery. Therefore, in order to complete the whole Fontan surgery in the future, the folded patch used for closure of the superior vena cava and right atrium connection should be removed through the right atrial incision, in addition to the implantation of the intracardiac lateral tunnel patch that connects the inferior vena cava to the pulmonary artery (Fig. 14.5).

Although Norwood's hemi-Fontan surgery can be completed using only one patch, it is difficult to determine the size, material, and shape of the patch, as well as how to suture it. Especially because the surgery is primarily the second operation in the staged surgical process, there is not a large enough autologous pericardial patch available, and allogeneic patch is hard to obtain. Modified hemi-Fontan surgery simplifies these difficulties. A patch of Gore-Tex material can be used in different sizes and thicknesses. There are generally three incisions. The incisions of the

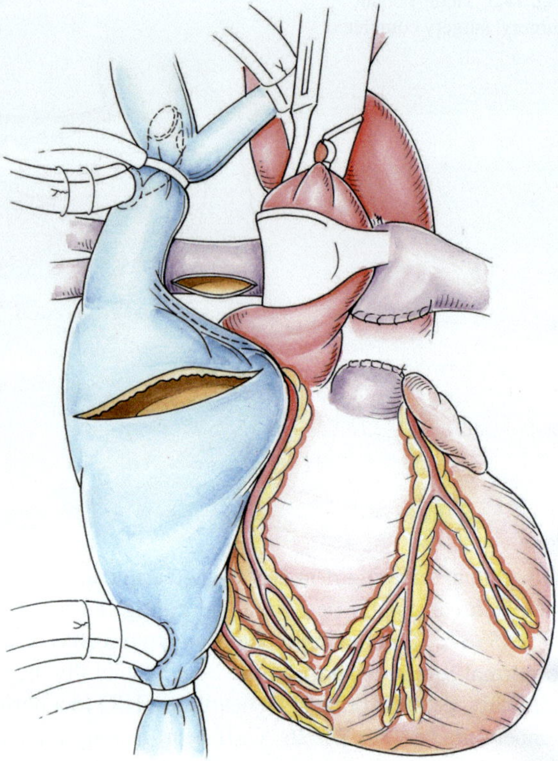

Fig. 14.6 Improved hemi-Fontan surgery: right atrium and pulmonary artery incision

right pulmonary artery and right atrium are available for the cavopulmonary channels; the upfront transverse incision of the right atrium is used to implant the separate patches (Fig. 14.6).

The transverse incision in the right pulmonary artery should be large. The size of the completed right atrium-pulmonary anastomosis should be twice the diameter of the superior vena cava. Opposite the right pulmonary artery incision, a right atrial transverse incision is made, extending from the right atrial end of the superior vena cava to the atrial appendage along the upper edge of the right atrial appendage, away from the sinoatrial node. The lower edge of the right pulmonary artery and rear edge of right atrial incision are continuously sutured together using 6-0 Prolene to construct the back wall of the cavopulmonary anastomosis, followed by the tightening and knotting of the suture ends. At this stage, the right atrial transverse incision is below the completed anastomosis. This transverse incision can also be an atrial septal resection (Fig. 14.7).

The materials of the patch used for closing the anterior wall of the anastomosis of the superior vena cava to right pulmonary artery can be varied according to the size of the anastomosis. The anastomosis is closed using continuous suturing. Through the transverse incision above the right atrium, the patch is sutured up to isolate the right atrium from superior vena cava. Different patch materials are available,

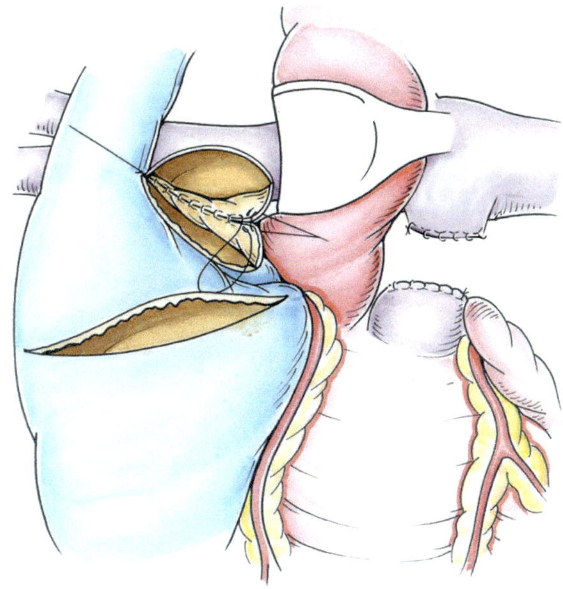

Fig. 14.7 Improved hemi-Fontan surgery: anastomosis of right atrium—pulmonary artery at posterior wall

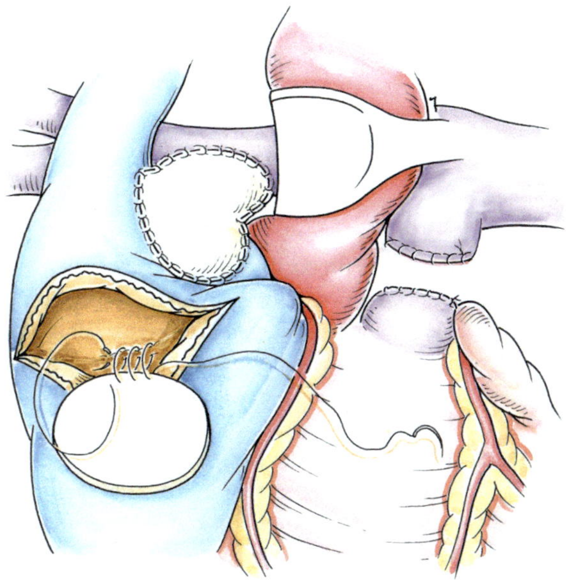

Fig. 14.8 Improved hemi-Fontan surgery: superior vena cava—pulmonary artery anastomosis closed, right atrium isolated from superior vena cava by patch

including both biological and Gore-Tex patches. The patch is placed at the conjunction of the superior vena cava and right atrium, the shape of which is round (Fig. 14.8). With the development of intervention technology, many surgeons consider biomaterial for the isolated patch during hemi-Fontan surgery; they believe that the total Fontan surgery can be performed through an intervention approach.

Fig. 14.9 Improved hemi-Fontan surgery: blood flow in superior vena cava after hemi-Fontan surgery

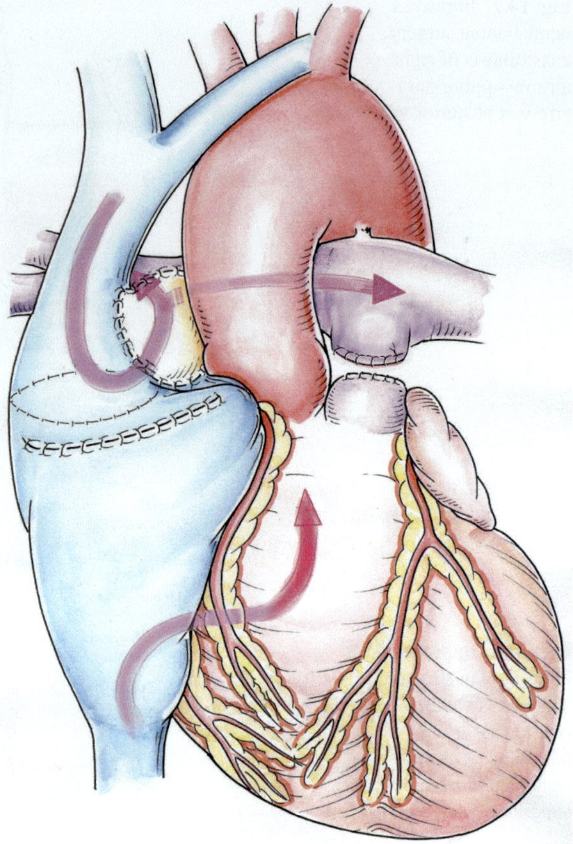

This figure shows blood flow after the separated patch has been set up. Superior vena caval blood flows into the left and right pulmonary arteries through the constructed anastomosis. The venous inferior vena caval blood mixed with systemic arterial blood flows into bodily circulation. The patch separates superior vena caval blood from the inferior vena cava (Fig. 14.9).

The final Fontan surgery of the total cavopulmonary connection can be implemented 6–12 months after the hemi-Fontan operation under cardiopulmonary bypass, at normal or low temperature, with routine use of cardioplegia after the aorta has been blocked. Superior and inferior vena caval cannulation should be adopted because the operation is performed in the atrium. In intra-atrium lateral tunnel Fontan surgery, the right atrial incision is located at the midline of the longitudinal axis of the inferior and superior vena cava, starting from the level of the atrium-separating patch from hemi-Fontan surgery, ending at the right atrium entrance of the inferior vena cava (Fig. 14.10).

The tricuspid valve or its traces, as well as a large atrial septal defect after removal of the atrial septum, can be seen after cutting the right atrium open. Left and right pulmonary veins can be probed through the atrial septal defect. The patch

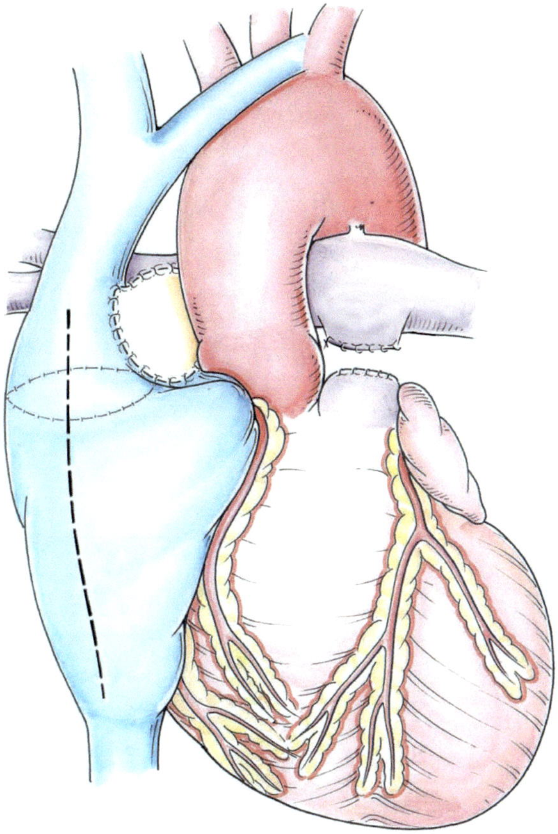

Fig. 14.10 Intra-atrium lateral tunnel Fontan surgery: right atrium incision

implanted by the hemi-Fontan procedure lies at the top of the right atrium, from which the superior vena cava is separated. If individually sewn in, the patch can be removed by removal of its sutures. Carefully check the patency of the superior vena cava and pulmonary artery anastomosis. Regarding a classic Norwood hemi-Fontan surgery in which a folded patch is used to separate the superior vena cava, careful attention should be paid to avoid cutting the continuous suture of the cavopulmonary anastomosis when removing the separating patch, resulting in anastomotic damage (Fig. 14.11).

In an intra-atrium lateral tunnel full Fontan operation, the side wall of the right atrium is used as part of a tunnel leading blood to the pulmonary artery, while the other side of the tunnel requires other materials. Surgeons often choose Gore-Tex artificial blood vessels, which are naturally shaped like a half-pipe after splitting them in half. A 4–6 mm hole is preset in the middle of the patch as a shunt between systemic venous and arterial flow to reduce pressure. Shaping both ends of patch like a semicircle aids in its suturing to the inferior and superior venae cavae without wrinkles. The location of the patch suturing is shown by the dotted line along the edges of the atrial septal defect, extending respectively to the junctions of the

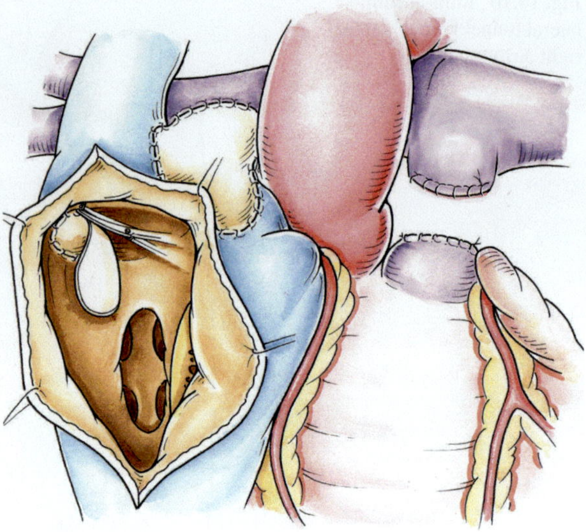

Fig. 14.11 Intra-atrium lateral tunnel Fontan surgery: removing the patch for isolation of the superior vena cava

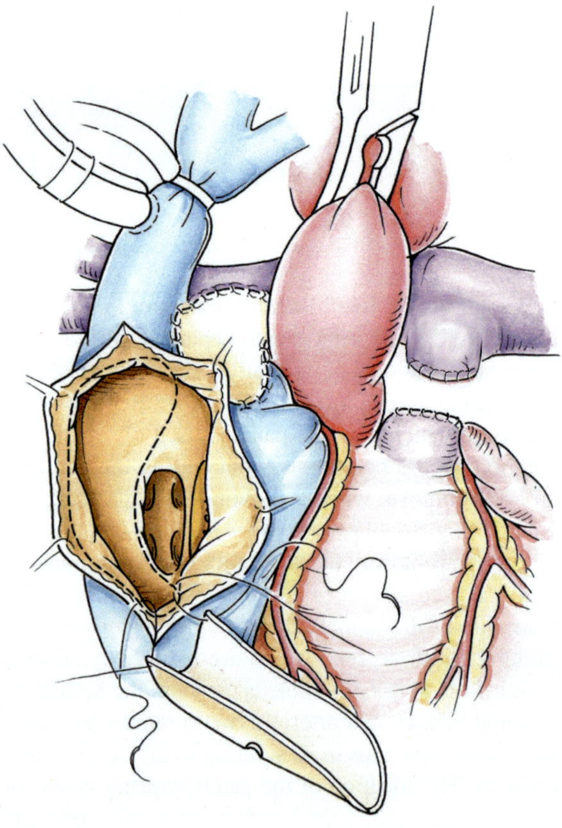

Fig. 14.12 Intra-atrium tunnel patch and its suture position

inferior and superior venae cavae with the right atrium. The diameter of lateral tunnel should be equivalent to approximately 150% of the diameter of the systemic vein. The suture is 5-0 Prolene (Fig. 14.12).

After the lateral tunnel has been established, blood of the superior vena cava flows to the right and left pulmonary arteries, as it did in the original hemi-Fontan surgery, while blood from the inferior vena cava also flows to right and left pulmonary arteries through the lateral tunnel. The right atrium is then closed by continuous suture (Fig. 14.13).

Notes From a conceptual standpoint, hemi-Fontan surgery is convenient for a subsequent full Fontan operation, and can also be performed with interventional therapy. However, hemi-Fontan surgery must be carried out under cardiopulmonary bypass, and the establishment of a Fontan intracardiac tunnel is also time-consuming and difficult. In contrast, bidirectional Glenn shunts do not require cardiopulmonary bypass, and the completion of full Fontan surgery with an extracardiac conduit is also simple.

Hemi-Fontan surgery and bidirectional Glenn shunts both act as intermediate palliation for a final total cavopulmonary connection—i.e., the total Fontan operation. The methods concerning the Fontan connection are summarized as follows:

1. Intracardiac lateral tunnel Fontan surgery (Fig. 14.13)
2. Intracardiac conduit Fontan surgery (Fig. 13.1)
3. Extracardiac conduit Fontan surgery (Fig. 15.1)
4. Extracardiac tunnel Fontan surgery (Fig. 15.4)

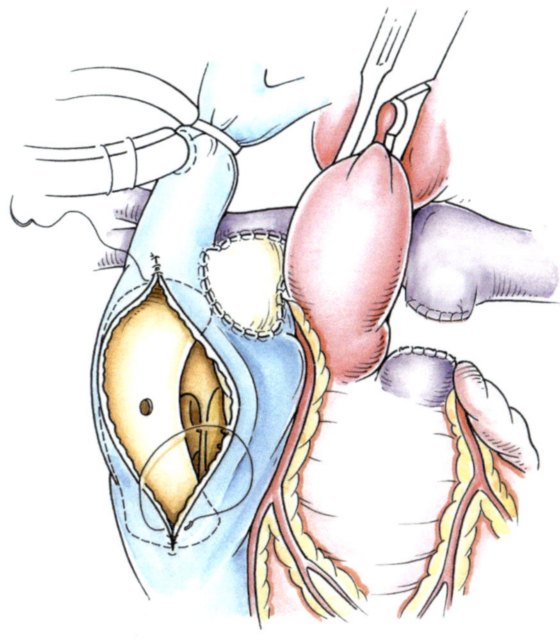

Fig. 14.13 Intra-atrium lateral tunnel constructed

Chapter 15
Extracardiac Conduit Full Fontan Surgery: Total Cavopulmonary Connection

Bin Qiao and Tong Jian Wang

Humes et al. formally performed the extracardiac conduit total cavopulmonary connection in 1988; Marcelletti subsequently reported and popularized this surgery (Marcelletti et al. 1990). The potential advantages of the extracardiac conduit total cavopulmonary connection are enumerated as follows: (1) normal atrial pressure is maintained; (2) the right atrium is bypassed, which reduces arrhythmia caused by an intra-atrial operation; (3) extracorporeal circulation at normal temperature with heart arrested or beating; (4) extracardiac conduit fenestration with no necessary extracorporeal circulation aid. Before the popularization of this surgery, functional single ventricle was treated mainly by an intra-atrium lateral tunnel total cavopulmonary connection. However, after 1988, and especially in the late 1990s, the use of the extracardiac conduit began to increase. A conduit made of Gore-Tex with a reinforcing ring was usually employed.

15.1 Gore-Tex Artificial Blood Vessel Extracardiac Conduit

The usage of Gore-Tex artificial blood vessels for an inferior vena cava-pulmonary artery anastomosis offers several advantages, likely including: (1) more uniform linear blood flow, as well as less turbulence and energy consumption; (2) lower risk of pulmonary venous return or atrioventricular valve obstruction. Without the potential of growth, artificial vessels should be larger than the inferior vena cava to delay and reduce reoperation occurrences. The appropriate diameter ratio of the artificial blood vessel to the inferior vena cava is 1.5:1. Too large a conduit can lead to

B. Qiao (✉) · T. J. Wang
Cardiovascular Institute, General Hospital of Jinan Military Region, Jinan, China

Cardiac surgery center, Western District of Shandong Provincial Hospital, Jinan, China

B. Qiao et al. (eds.), *Surgical Atlas of Functional Single Ventricle and Hypoplastic Left Heart Syndrome*, https://doi.org/10.1007/978-981-10-8435-5_15

turbulence and increased energy consumption. Therefore, an artificial blood vessel diameter of 18–22 mm is a generally appropriate size. An artificial blood vessel with a valve is rarely used today. Disadvantages of Gore-Tex conduit include: (1) no growth potential of the conduit; (2) the subsequent exclusion of younger patients; (3) prone to thrombosis formation in both the conduit and fenestration.

The operative procedure of using Gore-Tex artificial vasculature with reinforcing rings is simple. Gore-Tex sutures are usually adopted for suturing the inferior and superior vena caval anastomosis; however, Prolene sutures are another option. Because vena caval pressure is not high, blood leakage at the Gore-Tex pin hole can be stopped by compression hemostasis. Artificial blood vessels that are 1.5 times the diameter of the systemic vein are often suitable for the growth of a child for many years, even into adulthood. The two anastomoses of the right pulmonary artery to the superior and inferior venae cavae should be staggered with respect to each other in order to avoid flow collision of systemic venous blood upon its return to the pulmonary artery. This will affect pulmonary perfusion volume, and the staggered location will depend on anatomy and the convenience of the procedure. When a fenestration is performed between the Gore-Tex artificial vessel and the atrium, it is necessary to remove the reinforcement ring near the fenestration (Fig. 15.1).

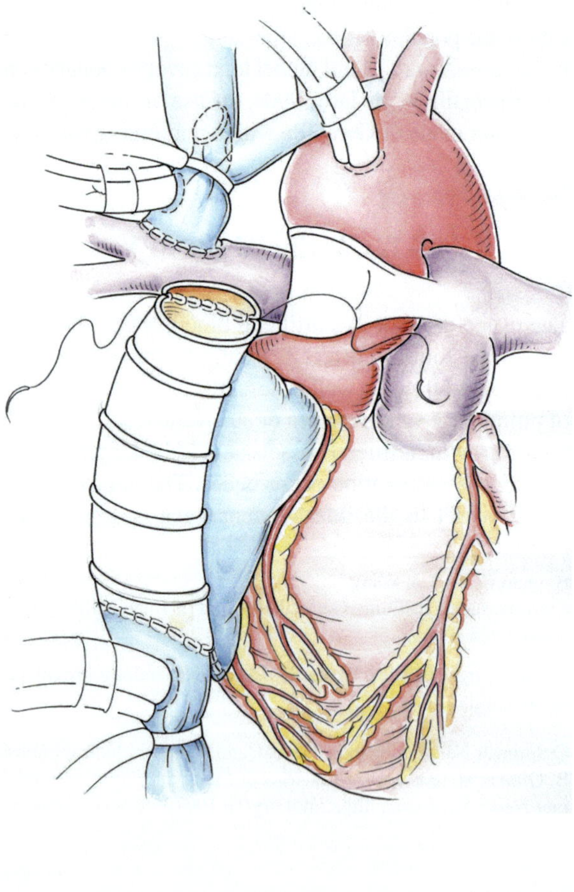

Fig. 15.1 Extracardiac conduit Fontan surgery: Gore-Tex artificial vascular with reinforcing ring

Artificial vessels made of other materials, such as Dacron, can also be used for the extracardiac conduit. Figure 15.2 shows that the cavopulmonary anastomosis is on the inner side, and the artificial vessel-pulmonary artery anastomosis is on the outer side.

15.2 Orthotropic Autogenous Extra-pericardium Conduit

Considering the absence of Gore-Tex growth potential, Hvass designed and used an autologous pericardium patch as an extracardiac conduit in a total cavopulmonary connection in 1992 (Hvass et al. 1992). He argued that this extracardiac conduit had the theoretical advantages of growth potential, low incidence of thrombosis, and resistance to infection. Subsequent studies have confirmed the growth potential of autogenous extra-pericardium conduits.

After splitting the sternum, a longitudinal incision is performed to open the pericardium as close as possible to the left side of the patient, followed by two parallel transverse incisions orthogonal to the lower and upper ends of the original longitudinal incision. The pericardial upper edge incision is at the level of the left and right pulmonary arteries, while the lower edge incision is at the inferior vena cava dia-

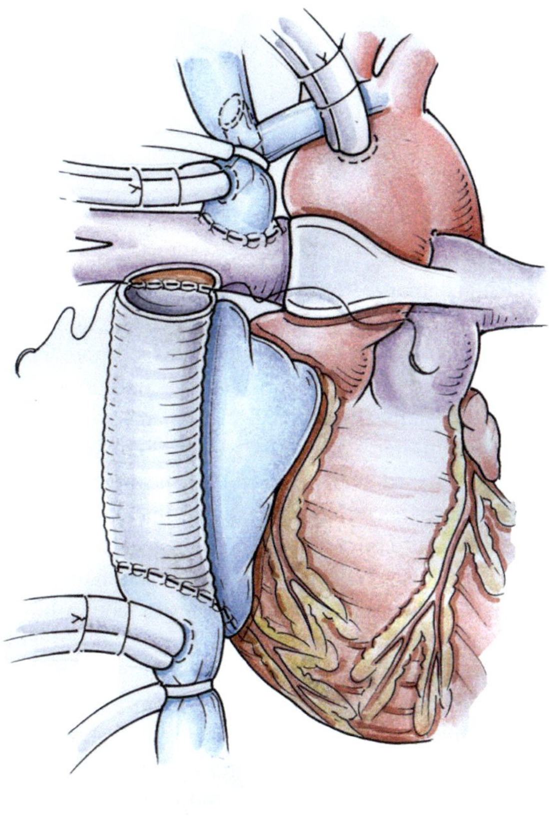

Fig. 15.2 Extracardiac conduit Fontan surgery: artificial vascular braided with polyester

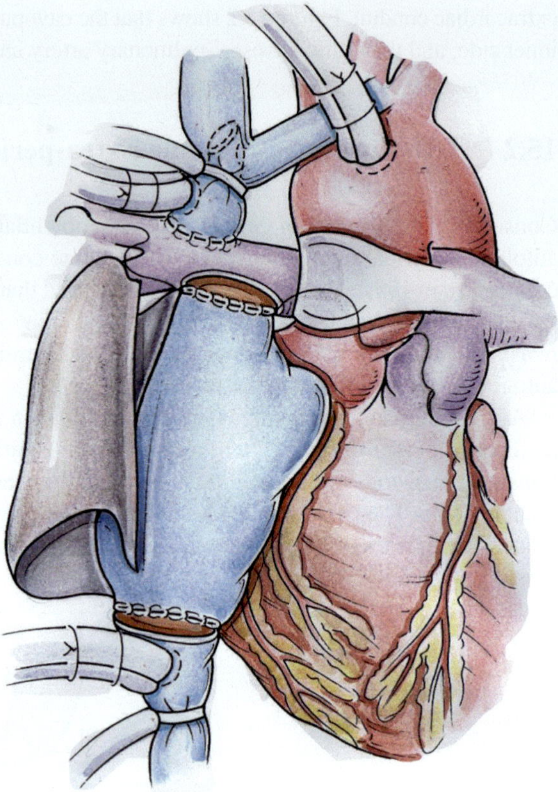

Fig. 15.3 In situ autologous pericardial conduit Fontan surgery: pericardium, right pulmonary artery semi-opening and inferior vena cava semi-opening

phragmatic level. Attention should be paid to the right phrenic nerve to avoid accidental damage. At this point, the cut pericardium has a left, upper, and lower free edge. After the pericardial flaps are ready, cannulation of the aorta, superior, and inferior venae cavae is performed. Extracorporeal circulation is established at normal temperature under heart-beating conditions. The superior vena cava is transected, and its distal end is end-to-side anastomosed with the upper lateral surface of the right pulmonary artery. Its proximal end is first sutured closed, and is then continuously sutured to the rear wall of the right pulmonary artery incision to be later used in the connection of the extracardiac conduit. The two cavopulmonary connection ports should be staggered with respect to each other to prevent blood flowing to pulmonary artery. It is only necessary to cut half of the junction between the inferior vena cava and right atrium at its anterior side, followed by the suturing of the right atrial-free anterior and posterior walls now attached to the inferior vena cava. At this point, the entire right atrium is bypassed, with the superior and inferior extremities of the right edge of the autologous pericardial flap facing the right pulmonary artery semi-opening and inferior vena cava semi-opening, respectively (Fig. 15.3).

The right atrium anterior lateral wall now becomes the posterior wall of the extracardiac conduit. The three free edges of the pericardium are continuously sutured with the pulmonary artery semi-opening, inferior vena cava semi-opening, and anterior wall

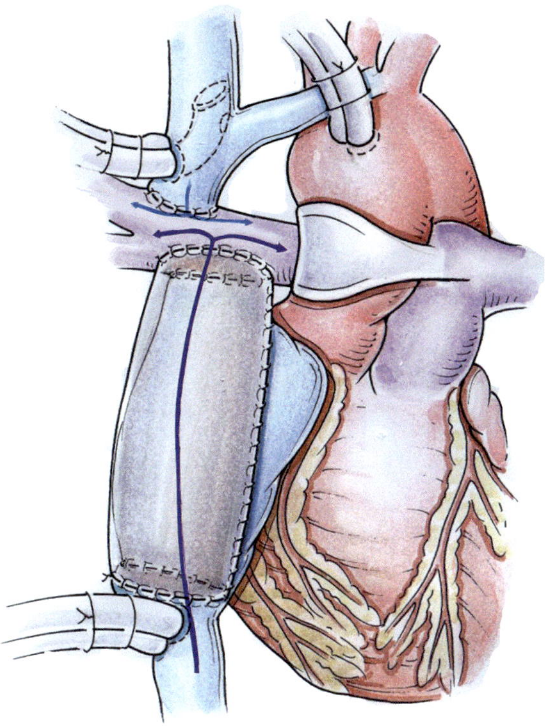

Fig. 15.4 Vena cava flow direction after autologous pericardial conduit Fontan surgery

of the right atrium, respectively. The blood flow direction of the pericardial extracardiac conduit Fontan connection is indicated in Fig. 15.4, and it can be seen that blood return from the inferior and superior venae cavae flows to the left and right pulmonary arteries, respectively, without colliding each other in the right pulmonary artery.

Notes The application of autogenous pericardium conduit in a Fontan connection may introduce some risks: (1) much of the suturing at the right atrium anterior wall may increase the post-operative risk of atrial flutter; (2) mobilization of the pericardial flap carries the risk of damaging the phrenic nerve; (3) pressure elevation of the extracardiac conduit would contribute to obstruction of pulmonary vein at the same side. Due to the presence of these risks, the instability of long-term efficacy, and much required effort for the suturing of the right atrial surface, this technique has not been widely promoted.

References

Hvass U, Pansard Y, Bohm G, Depoix J, Enguerrand D, Worms A. Bicaval pulmonary connection in tricuspid atresia using an extracardiac tube of autologous pediculated pericardium to bridge inferior vena cava. Eur J Cardiothorac. 1992;6(1):49–51. https://doi.org/10.1016/1010-7940(92)90099-j.

Marcelletti C, Corno A, Giannico S, Marino B. Inferior vena cava-pulmonary artery extracardiac conduit. A new form of right heart bypass. J Thorac Cardiovasc Surg. 1990;100(2):228–32.

Chapter 16
Intra-atrial Lateral Tunnel versus Extracardiac Conduit and Fenestrated Total Cavopulmonary Connection

Bin Qiao and Zheng Xiang Wang

Over the past two decades, the two methods named in the title of this chapter have been used to treat a large number of patients with functional single ventricle. Early mortality rates, early and mid-term postoperation hemodynamics, cardiac function, and complications have not been shown to be significantly different. As mentioned in earlier chapters, in intra-atrial lateral tunnel Fontan procedures, the lateral tunnel has the potential to grow, so it can be performed at any age, achieve excellent hemodynamics, and reduce atrial enlargement caused by increasing venous pressure. On the other hand, despite the lack of conduit growth ability, the extracardiac conduit Fontan procedure has shown similar hemodynamics. The operative technique is simple. It can be performed even without the support of extracorporeal circulation, or with beating heart conditions under extracorporeal circulation. This avoids most operation on the atrial surface thereby decreasing the risk of arrhythmia (Katogi 2012; Robbers-Visser et al. 2010). The long-term efficacy of this method has been proven to be excellent by nearly ten years of follow-up results. The early mortality rates of the two methods lie between 2 and 13%, with no significant difference between the two. At present, most scholars acknowledge that the extracardiac conduit Fontan surgery is a promising procedure that demonstrates lower ventricular resistance and energy loss but can only be applied to older children or adults, considering that the extracardiac conduit has no growth ability. On the contrary, the intra-atrial lateral tunnel total Fontan surgery is used in young children.

In the past, patients with increased pulmonary vascular resistance and mild to moderate heart insufficiency were Fontan surgery contraindications. An intra-atrial lateral tunnel fenestration or small extracardiac conduit atrial shunt affords the opportunity for these patients to undergo Fontan surgery. This technique places a

B. Qiao (✉) · Z. X. Wang
Cardiovascular Institute, General Hospital of Jinan Military Region, Jinan, China

Cardiac surgery center, Western District of Shandong Provincial Hospital, Jinan, China

B. Qiao et al. (eds.), *Surgical Atlas of Functional Single Ventricle and Hypoplastic Left Heart Syndrome*, https://doi.org/10.1007/978-981-10-8435-5_16

right-to-left shunt through the defect, filling the functional single ventricle in the diastolic period and thus maintaining adequate cardiac output. However, the cost of such a fenestration or shunt is the reduction of systemic oxygen saturation due to the reduction of pulmonary blood flow, which results from increased systemic blood volume and reduced vena caval pressure. Interventional treatment, which has been widely carried out, facilitated the fenestration operation as well as saved the trouble of considering the closure of fenestration in future. When the shunt or fenestration is no longer needed, it can be reduced or closed at any time by means of intervention. A disadvantage of this technique is the likelihood of local thrombosis formation.

A fenestration operation for an intra-atrial lateral tunnel Fontan procedure has already been planned preoperatively. After the intra-atrial lateral tunnel patch has been chosen, a hole of 4–5 mm in diameter is cut in the center of the patch. Because the patches are often made of Gore-Tex and other artificial materials, the hole should be cut using scissors to ensure that it is a smooth circle without any rough edges to avoid thrombosis formation. With the establishment of the atrial medial tunnel, the

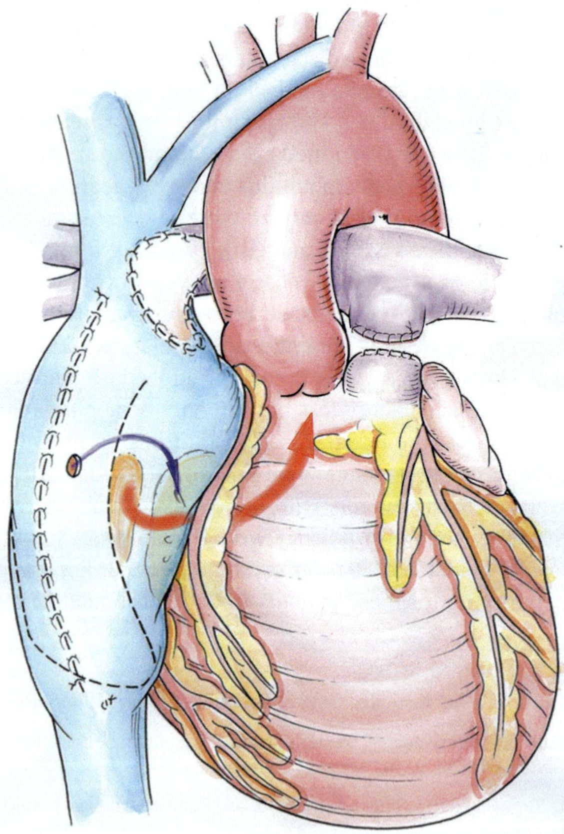

Fig. 16.1 Fenestration operation in intra-atrial tunnel Fontan

decompression of vena cava pressure is available with a right-to-left shunt through this hole, provided that vena caval pressure is too high (Fig. 16.1).

The fenestration operation is also determined preoperatively in patients who will undergo the extracardiac conduit Fontan surgery. Fenestration should be performed before weaning the patient off of cardiopulmonary bypass. Following the direct opening of a 5 mm hole 5 mm in both the extracardiac conduit and the corresponding position on the right atrial wall, either continuous suturing is performed, or an artificial vessel also 5 mm in diameter is placed between them. If the need for fenestration has not been identified before surgery, and pulmonary artery pressure is persistently sustained above 20 mmHg while weaning cardiopulmonary bypass, a hole has to be cut at off-pump with only artificial blood vessels available. Again, blood flow in a high-pressure vena cava can be shunted through the artificial vessel and the atrial septal defect into the left atrium (Fig. 16.2).

The fenestration can remain open if systemic oxygen saturation is maintained around 80%; it must be immediately closed through the intervention method if it persistently drops below 75%. The fenestration of either the intra-atrial lateral tunnel Fontan or extracardiac conduit Fontan can be occluded by the interventional technique.

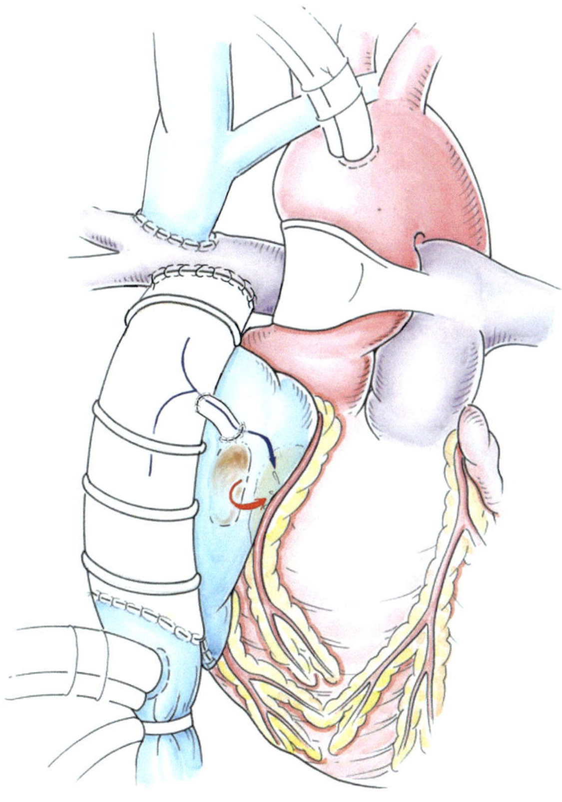

Fig. 16.2 Fenestration operation in extracardiac conduit Fontan

References

Katogi T. Extracardiac conduit Fontan procedure versus intra-atrial lateral tunnel Fontan procedure. Gen Thorac Cardiovasc Surg. 2012;60(12):792.

Robbers-Visser D, Miedema M, Nijveld A, Boersma E, Bogers AJJC, Haas F, Helbing WA, Kapusta L. Results of staged total cavopulmonary connection for functionally univentricular hearts; comparison of intra-atrial lateral tunnel and extracardiac conduit. Eur J Cardiothorac. 2010;37(4):934–41. https://doi.org/10.1016/j.ejcts.2009.10.016.

Chapter 17
New Concepts of Dynamic Fontan Surgery

Bin Qiao and Li Li Wu

For decades, the Fontan surgery forming the total cavopulmonary connection, designed for the treatment of functional single ventricles, had reduced operative mortality rates, improving long-term survival to the point that some patients live until adulthood. However, the Fontan surgery is ultimately a palliative procedure. A single anatomical ventricle, as a functional left ventricle, can sustain systemic circulation. With the right atrium being bypassed for the purpose of separating arteriovenous blood flow, the driving force for the entire venous return to pulmonary circulation is only dependent on the weak blood pressure of the superior vena cava and pulmonary artery. These abnormal hemodynamics cannot meet the normal physiological requirements of the human body, gradually leading to a series of pathological changes, such as changes in pulmonary circulation resistance, long-term chronic venous congestion, increased venous pressure, pleural fluid due to excessive exudate, ascites, edema, hypoproteinemia, heart failure, arrhythmia, hypoxemia, low cardiac output, thrombosis, etc. as well as to the formation of a so-called total cavopulmonary artery dysfunction, also known as Failing Fontan. The lack of a power source in the Fontan circulation can contribute to Failing Fontan, as well as to a variety of subsequent complications. Unless a heart transplant is performed promptly, other clinical treatments are rendered ineffective. Fontan surgery only solves the problem of arteriovenous blood separation in functional single ventricle. The new concept of power Fontan surgery aims to establish a more stable "biventricular physiology" by mechanically supporting the Fontan circulation, allowing the inherent single ventricle to continue to exert left ventricular

B. Qiao (✉)
Cardiovascular Institute, General Hospital of Jinan Military Region, Jinan, China

Cardiac Surgery Center, Western District of Shandong Provincial Hospital, Jinan, China

L. L. Wu
Institute of Cardiovascular Diseases, Jinan Military Region General Hospital of PLA, Jinan, China

B. Qiao et al. (eds.), *Surgical Atlas of Functional Single Ventricle and Hypoplastic Left Heart Syndrome*, https://doi.org/10.1007/978-981-10-8435-5_17

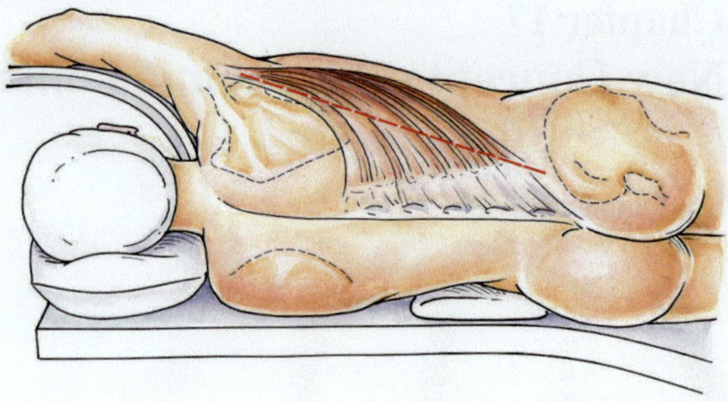

Fig. 17.1 Dynamic Fontan surgery: the incision of latissimus dorsi muscle

function and the mechanically assisted Fontan circulation to work as the "right ventricle" function. Since mechanical assist devices have been widely applied in the clinic to treat end-stage heart failure since the late 1980s, some surgeons have tried to adopt mechanical assist devices as temporary approaches to deal with Failing Fontan while their patients wait for heart transplantation. Permanent mechanical assistance available for Fontan circulation has not been reported in the clinic at present. To understand the new concept of dynamic Fontan surgery, several factors relating to the mechanical assist device should be considered: (1) permanent power; (2) extracardiac implantation, therefore suitable for extracardiac conduit Fontan surgery; (3) one-way direction circulation; (4) power at the cavopulmonary level; (5) pulsation and synchronization with heart rate; (6) pressure range of 0–30 mmHg. The dozens of mechanical assist devices already presented in practice are hardly suitable in the overall design of a dynamic Fontan surgery.

According the editor's imagination, a dynamic Fontan surgery driven by the latissimus dorsi is described below.

The latissimus dorsi muscle is one of the largest and most powerful skeletal muscles in body and is triangular in shape. The right latissimus dorsi attaches to the right scapula on one end, and to the right side of the spine on its bottom side, leaving its two lateral sides free. Patients are placed in a left-lateral supine position in surgery with their right side facing up and right hand abducted. The incision is made from the right scapula of the right shoulder obliquely to the upper edge of the right ilium (Fig. 17.1).

Generally, the latissimus dorsi can be clearly exposed after incising the skin and dissecting subcutaneous fat. Not attached by any muscle fibers, the free edge of the latissimus dorsi, with only a few membranes connected to the surrounding tissue, can be easily separated away. All arterial and venous blood supply, as well as the nerves dominating the latissimus dorsi, come from the muscle's attachment point at the scapula, traveling deeply into the muscular layer. Great care should be taken not to damage nerves and blood vessels during latissimus dorsi separation. The edge of the latissimus dorsi attached to the spine, which is only comprised of tendon and not muscle fibers, can be sharply dissected. A small part of the edge of the latissimus dorsi attached to the ilium can also be cut from the ilium. The whole latissimus dorsi with its muscular pedicle is shown (Fig. 17.2).

The two pacemaker leads with suture needles are now sutured at the pedicle end of the latissimus dorsi muscle, away from the nerves and blood vessels which should

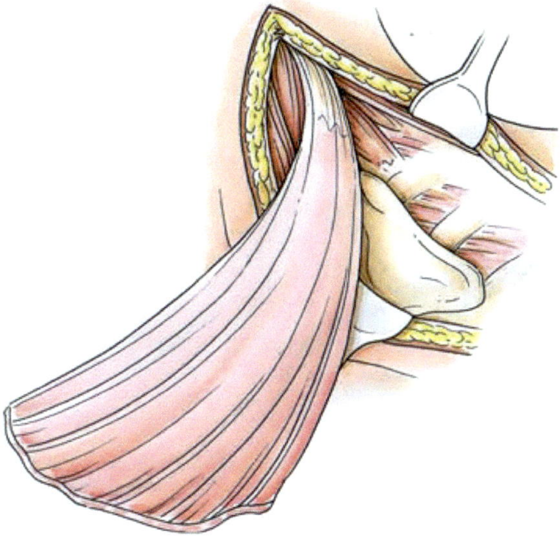

Fig. 17.2 Dynamic Fontan surgery: dissecting latissimus dorsi muscle

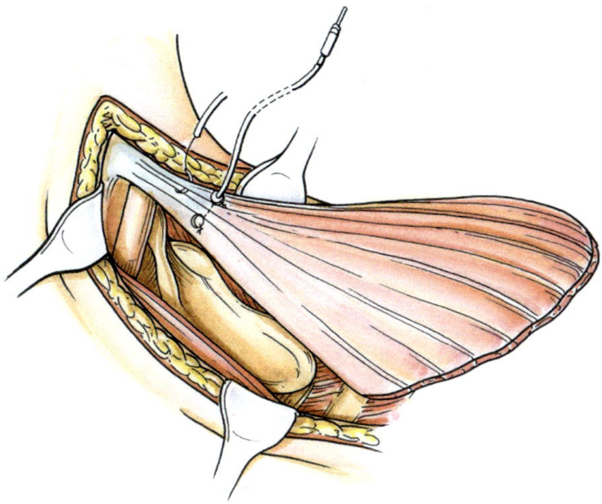

Fig. 17.3 Dynamic Fontan Surgery: suturing pacing wires

be carefully identified first. The two leads apart 1 cm from each other. After the suture needles cut off, they should be very tightly fixed to the latissimus dorsi by using silicone pads and Prolene at the two sites where the leads pass into and out of the muscle. Because the muscle fibers are not cut off, the latissimus dorsi could be perfectly preserved as a whole. Therefore, bleeding is seldom found even though the wound is large (Fig. 17.3).

A 4–5 cm transverse incision is made in the second intercostal at the midclavicular line, and approximately 4 cm of the second rib is removed. The latissimus dorsi with pedicle and two pacemaker leads are placed in the right thoracic cavity through a subcutaneous tunnel (Fig. 17.4).

Fig. 17.4 Dynamic Fontan Surgery: placing latissimus dorsi and pacemaker wires in right thoracic cavity

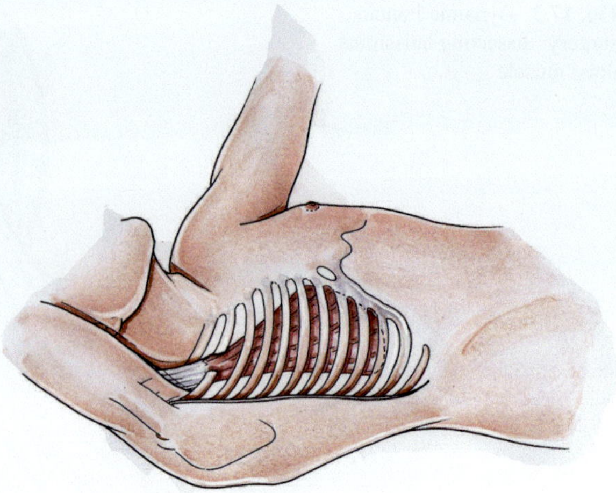

Fig. 17.5 Dynamic Fontan surgery: fixing latissimus dorsi muscle

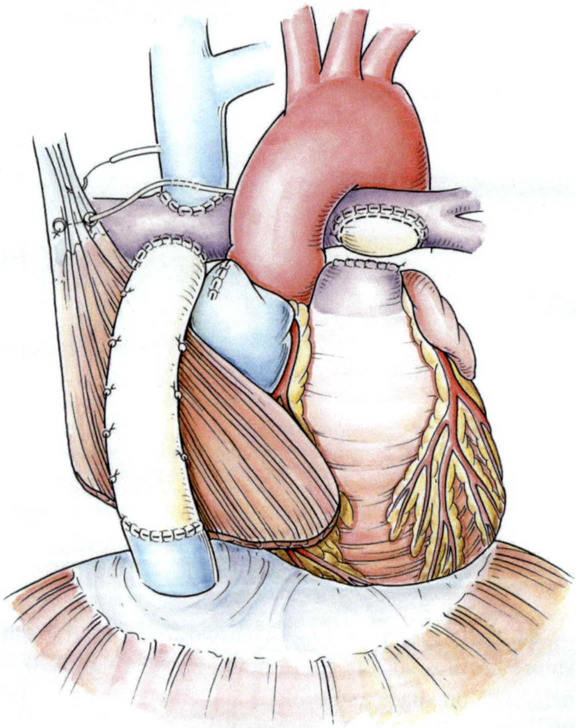

Figure 17.5 shows a completed Fontan connection with the total extracardiac conduit directly connected to the inferior vena cava and right pulmonary artery. The latissimus dorsi is placed smoothly in the right thoracic cavity behind the extracardiac conduit. The latissimus dorsi is anastomosed to the extracardiac conduit at

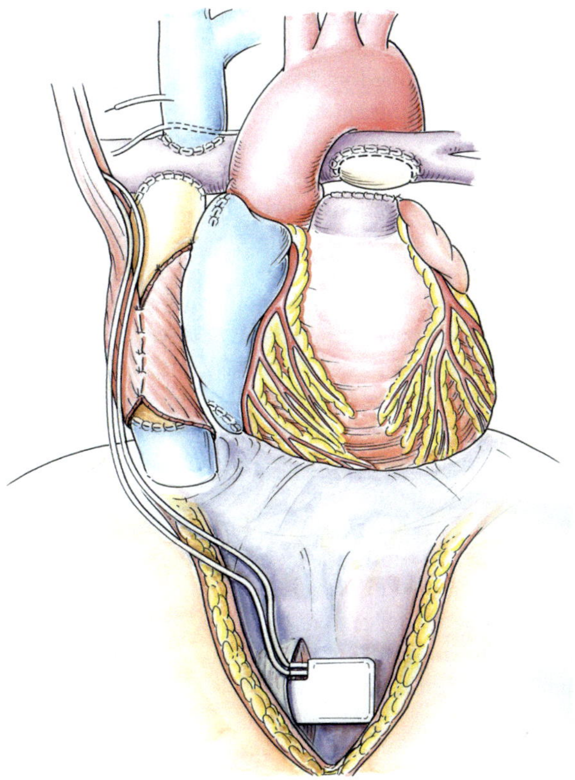

Fig. 17.6 Dynamic Fontan surgery: connecting pacing wire with pacemaker

several sites on both sides with interrupted Prolene and fixed by tying knots to avoid slipping when the latissimus dorsi muscle contracts.

With the latissimus dorsi wrapping around the extracardiac conduit in the total Fontan surgery, its two free edges are tightly sutured together to ensure a close fit. Two pacing wires are connected to a pacemaker, which is embedded in the right rectus abdominis sheath through a middle chest incision. A unipolar VVI pacemaker is adopted, which can be adjusted according to the patient's inherent heart rate. The latissimus dorsi will contract when stimulated by the pacemaker's electrical pulses synchronized with the heart rate and will subsequently squeeze the extracardiac conduit to produce the power to pump at least the inferior vena caval blood into the pulmonary artery. The superior vena caval return to the pulmonary artery still rely on the weak pressure gradient between the superior vena cava and pulmonary artery. As long as the cavopulmonary anastomosis and conduit-pulmonary anastomosis are not in a line, most of the inferior vena caval blood will be conducted to the pulmonary artery (Fig. 17.6).

Notes In the 1980s, Carpentier, a French doctor, proposed the idea that cardiac function failure could be mechanically assisted by latissimus dorsi muscle wrapped around the entire ventricle. With numerous animal tests and laboratory studies, supported and promoted by the company Medtronic, the project obtained the permission of the European Community Drug Administration for clinical trials. A synchronization training of the latissimus with the heart was performed using a pacemaker modified by Medtronic to increase cardiac output. Three months later, synchronized contraction with the heart rate was achieved. Although there were many positive clinical reports at that time, in 1989, the authors carried it out on six cases in the clinic with a lack of effective results. All patients underwent the placement of latissimus dorsi muscle around their hearts, but all of the latissimus trainings were not completed within three months due to acute heart failure. They later underwent either implantation of mechanical heart aids or heart transplants in place of the latissimus dorsi. Indeed, the latissimus dorsi may show a strong contraction under electric pulse stimulation; however, it cannot immediately reach a synchronized systole and diastole with the heart after wrapping around it, and the exhausted heart cannot endure the training for three months either. Additionally, during diastole the contraction of the latissimus dorsi muscle further reduced the diastolic volume, reducing cardiac output, and resulting in deteriorating heart failure. Fortunately, the muscle only exerts a contractile function in total Fontan surgery, so the synchronization issue is no longer a concern. Furthermore, systolic pressure can reach up to 30 mmHg. This might be promising approach in total Fontan surgery. One-way flow achievement will be the vital problem that could potentially be resolved by the placement of two venous valves in the superior and inferior venae cavae. The implantation of the venous valves should be simple, lacking the need for anticoagulation with a durable valve.

Chapter 18
Pulsating Balloon Assisted Fontan Surgery's Total Cavopulmonary Circulation

Bin Qiao, Li Li Wu, and Yi Yan Jiang

Among hundreds of cardiac mechanical assist devices, the application of an intra-aortic balloon pump or ascending aortic balloon to support extracardiac conduit Fontan circulation is another new concept that can improve the power source of Fontan surgery. Two extracardiac balloons are placed around short superior vena caval and extracardiac conduits, which are powered by an intra-aortic balloon counterpulsation machine. They can synchronously expand or contract to squeeze blood from the superior and inferior venae cavae into the pulmonary artery.

The superior vena cava balloon capacity is approximately 15 mL, shaped like an oval, and 15 mm in diameter; the extracardiac conduit balloon capacity is 40 mL, also shaped like an oval, and is 5 mm in diameter. Each balloon is made of durable synthetic silica gel and is tightly adhered on the left of a Dacron patch that will later be used to wrap the superior vena cava or extracardiac conduit. To facilitate Dacron patch with balloon passing through the superior vena cava and extracardiac conduit, balloon opposite side Dacron patch can be completely reserved, upper and lower ends of the Dacron patch being cut, the edge of balloon side Dacron patch being left. After being tightly wrapped around the superior vena cava and extracardiac conduit, the two edges of the patch are sutured together. The two balloons are connected with a silicone tube to inflate and deflate them, the other end of which is connected to the intra-aortic balloon pump. The intra-aortic balloon pump widely used in the clinic today can provide a maximal inflated volume of 60 mL, which is enough for the inflation of the two balloons. The main machine, also known as the controller, can

B. Qiao (✉)
Cardiovascular Institute, General Hospital of Jinan Military Region, Jinan, China

Cardiac Surgery Center, Western District of Shandong Provincial Hospital, Jinan, China

L. L. Wu · Y. Y. Jiang
Institute of Cardiovascular Diseases Jinan Military Region General Hospital of PLA, Jinan, China

B. Qiao et al. (eds.), *Surgical Atlas of Functional Single Ventricle and Hypoplastic Left Heart Syndrome*, https://doi.org/10.1007/978-981-10-8435-5_18

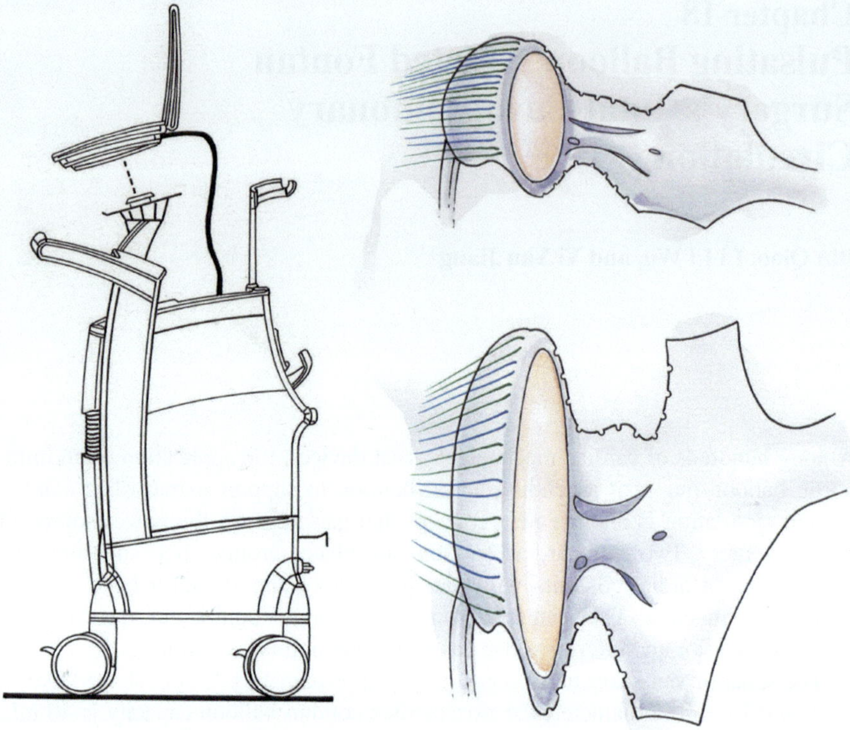

Fig. 18.1 Fontan circulation assisted by balloon pump: balloon and counterpulsation device

provide power for balloon counterpulsation as well as a computer screen showing electrocardiogram, blood pressure, working state, etc. Balloon pulsation is synchronized with the heartbeat based on the patient's Q-wave from ECG or a pacemaker rhythm (Fig. 18.1).

This figure shows total Fontan surgery using an extracardiac conduit for a functional single ventricle case, in which the pulmonary artery has been transected and its two ends closed. Balloon pulsation-assisted Fontan circulation can be simultaneously performed after completion of the extracardiac conduit anastomosis during the Fontan surgery. Only concerning the extracardiac operation, it is recommended to perform this procedure when weaning cardiopulmonary bypass with all intubation removed and protamine neutralizing heparin. The small balloon is placed around the superior vena cava directly below the innominate vein, while the large balloon is positioned around the conduit and the inferior vena cava near the diaphragm. Because the balloon and ventilation ducts are connected together, the two balloons are placed on the right side of what they encircle. After the Dacron with a balloon has been wrapped tightly around the superior vena cava and extracardiac conduit, the gas in the balloon is drawn out. The interrupted sutures previously placed on the Dacron patch can be pulled out by piercing the opposite edge of the patch, its two ends being knotted. Any redundant patch is cut away. To prevent the patch from slipping, its upper and lower ends should be fixed on the conduit, inferior, and superior venae cavae using additional knotted sutures (Fig. 18.2).

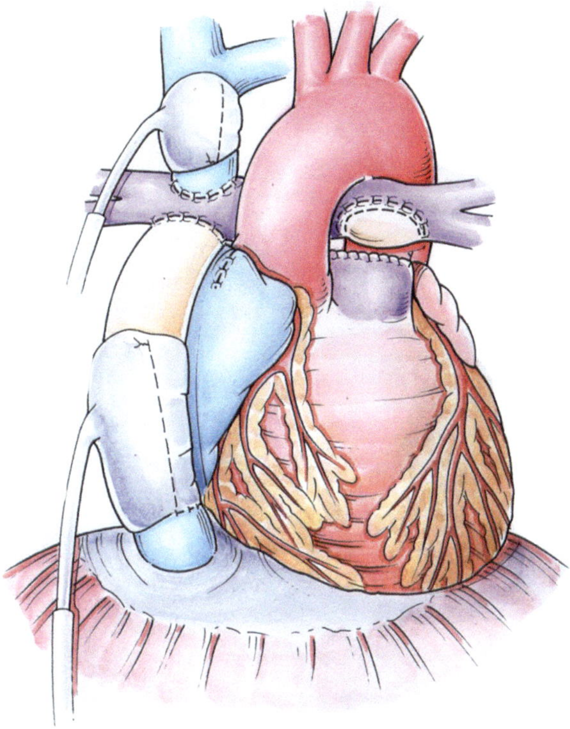

Fig. 18.2 Fontan circulation assisted by balloon pump: balloon wrapped outside the extracardiac conduit and superior vena cava

The subcutaneous and out-of-skin segments of the silicone ventilation tube that connects the balloons are covered with another Dacron patch. This patch can help the ventilation tube and the subcutaneous tissue to closely stick together and to prevent retrograde infection from spreading along the tube. A small incision, the same size as the tube, is made in the skin at the lower right 4 cm of the umbilicus. The ventilation tube wrapped with polyester is pulled out from skin incision under the right costal arch through the pericardial cavity with long curved forceps and fixed with sutures. After entered the incision, the forceps travel subcutaneously from outside to inside, from bottom to top, and penetrate the abdominal muscles under the rib arch (Fig. 18.3).

The ventilation tube is connected with an intra-aortic balloon pump. After the counterpulsation machine and ECG leads have been connected, the balloon will inflate and empty with the heart beating. Figure 18.4 shows that inferior and superior vena caval blood flows to the pulmonary artery when the balloon empties.

When the balloon inflates, inferior and superior vena caval blood is simultaneously squeezed into the pulmonary artery. The upper and lower balloons serve as valves to prevent forward-moving systemic blood from flowing backwards. Because the lung is a ventilation organ, pulmonary arterial blood already present in the alveoli is not likely to return to the pulmonary artery. Negative pressure formed when the balloons deflate is conducive to the return of systemic venous blood to the pulmonary artery (Fig. 18.5).

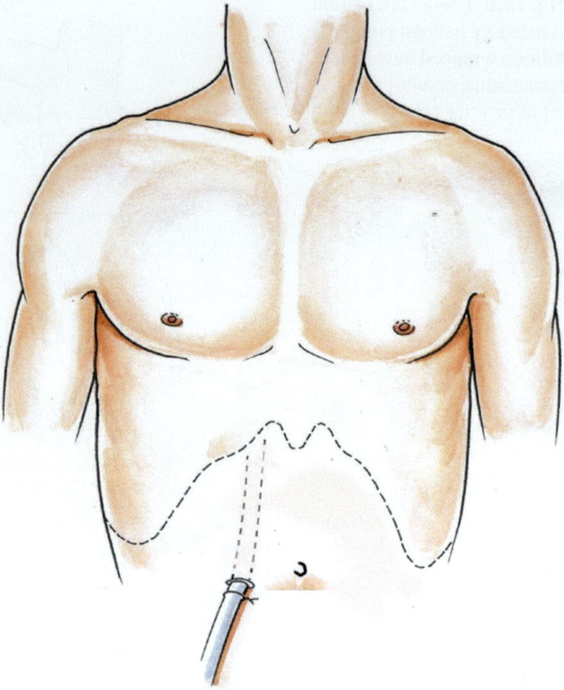

Fig. 18.3 Balloon assisted Fontan cycle: ventilation duct implantation and fixation

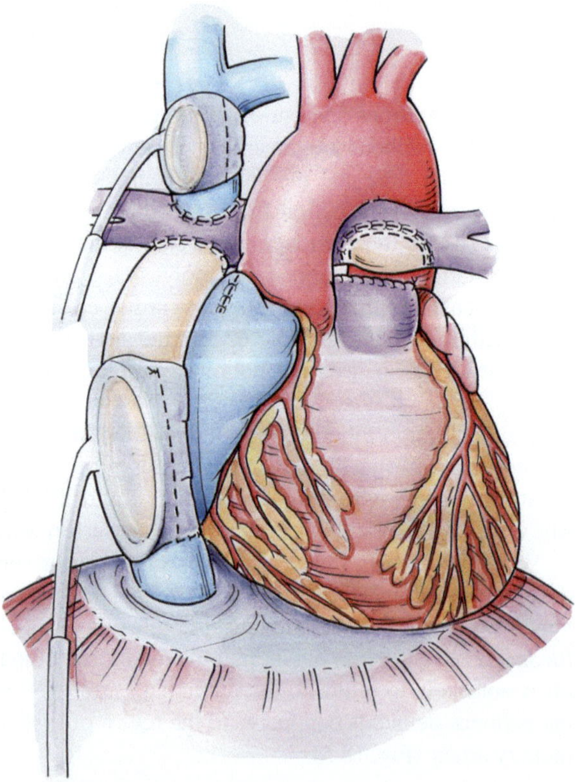

Fig. 18.4 Balloon assisted Fontan cycle: balloon emptying state

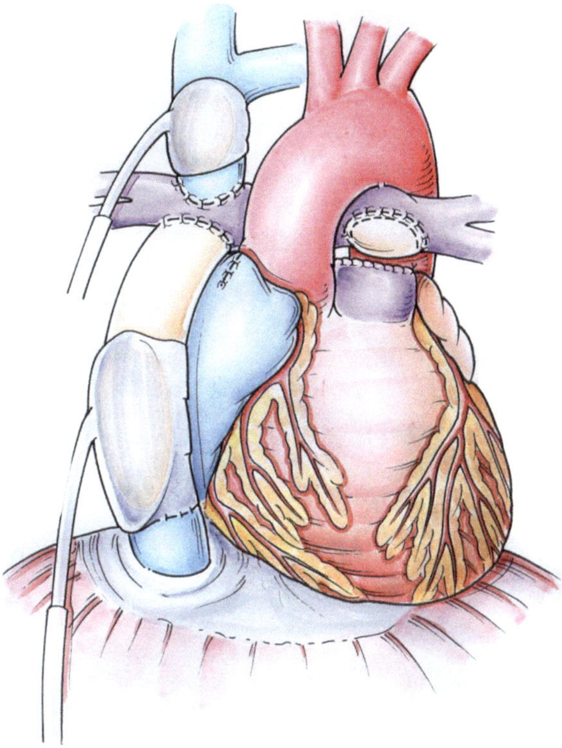

Fig. 18.5 Balloon assisted Fontan cycle: balloon filling state

C-Pulse is a mechanical circulatory assist device designed by the American company Sunshine, specifically to treat patients with Class III chronic heart failure, as defined by the American Heart Association. The machine is currently in a period of clinical trials. The authors proposed the idea of applying C-Pulse as a driving force in the Fontan operation to the company's engineers. However, because extra-aortic balloon pulsation devices are initially designed for adults, they must be redesigned as a power source for Fontan surgery. Additionally, if only a single balloon is wrapped around the extracardiac conduit, additional valves should be placed in the inferior and superior venae cavae to prevent backflow of blood during balloon inflation. As a result, surgery time and operation difficulty would increase, and there are many additional problems related to valve placement, such as anticoagulation and the durability of the valves. Therefore, two balloons are employed to act as valves; one is wrapped around the superior vena cava, and another around the extracardiac conduit. The required maximum pulse pressure is lower than pulmonary artery systolic pressure, so 30 mmHg is sufficient. In order to synchronize the balloons with the heartbeat, two beat-sensitive electrodes are installed on the surface of the heart during surgery. The electrode power lines, along with the ventilation duct, are connected by an adapter to a portable controller battery that can work continuously for at least 8 h after a charge. Figure 18.6 shows an ideal design. Emerging from the right lower abdomen, two cardiac surface electrodes and the balloon ventilation duct are connected to the battery and controller, respectively; patients can freely carry these devices with them.

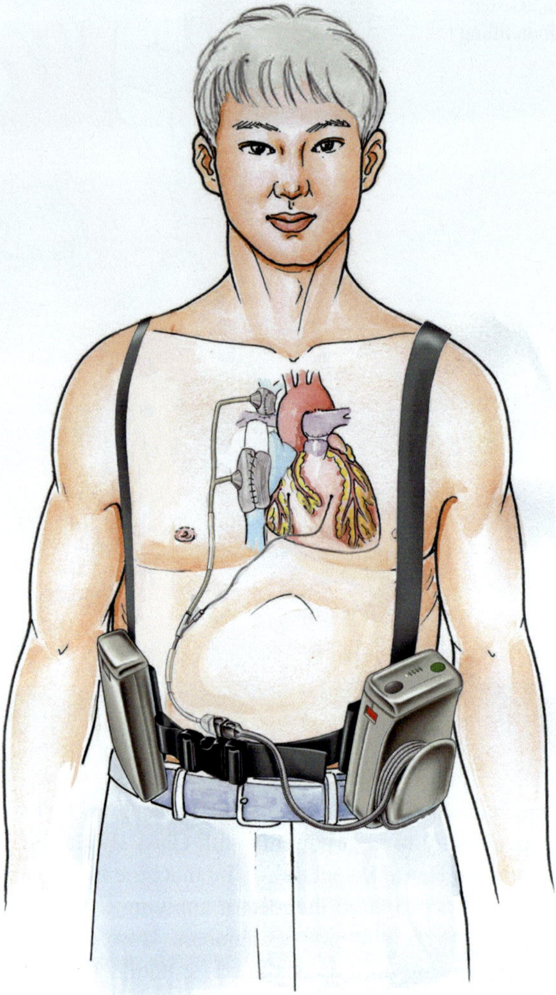

Fig. 18.6 Fontan circulation assist device developed by Sunshine company

Part II
Hypoplastic Left Heart Syndrome

Chapter 19
Basic Conception

Yu Guo Weng and Bin Qiao

Hypoplastic left heart syndrome (HLHS), also known as left ventricular hypoplasia syndrome, is a group of complex congenital heart diseases involving left ventricular, aortic, aortic valve, and mitral valve hypoplasia, as well as other derived deformations that need to maintain systemic and pulmonary circulation. The main lesions of HLHS include a small ascending aorta and aortic arch, as well as aortic stenosis or atresia, which can be combined with mitral stenosis or atresia; the left ventricle is inadequately developed and has no function, often combined with endocardial elastic fiber hyperplasia continuous with the mitral valve. Generally, the left atrium is smaller than normal, and the atrial wall is thicker, often associated with an atrial septal defect or patent foramen ovale, which acts as major sources of oxygenated blood for the right ventricle. Therefore, it is more appropriate to name it hypoplastic left ventricle syndrome. In order to sustain systemic and pulmonary circulation, the right ventricle is required to pump blood not only to the pulmonary artery, but also to the aorta through the patent ductus arteriosus. Excessive overload of the right heart can contribute to enlargement or hypertrophy of the right atrium and right ventricle, while abnormally enlarging the pulmonary artery trunk and left and right pulmonary arteries.

HLHS is most common as a congenital heart disease in Europe and the United States, with incidence among patients less than one-year-old reported to be between 7% and 9%. Due to the complexity and severity of the deformity, patients often die

Y. G. Weng (✉)
German Heart Center (Berlin), Berlin, Germany
e-mail: wengyuguo@dhzb.de

B. Qiao
Cardiovascular Institute, General Hospital of Jinan Military Region, Jinan, China

Cardiac Surgery Center, Western District of Shandong Provincial Hospital, Jinan, China

B. Qiao et al. (eds.), *Surgical Atlas of Functional Single Ventricle and Hypoplastic Left Heart Syndrome*, https://doi.org/10.1007/978-981-10-8435-5_19

within a few hours or days after birth if intervention is not taken as soon as possible; unless correct diagnosis and appropriate treatments have been made and performed in an experienced congenital heart disease treatment center, children rarely survive the neonatal period. At present, routine perinatal and postnatal neonatal echocardiography diagnoses have not been popularized in China, so there are no accurate incidence statistics. According to German Congenital Heart Disease Association statistics from 2010, HLHS accounted for 1–2% of congenital heart disease in Germany, of which two-thirds of the cases were male. In a report from the US Center for Disease Control and Prevention (CDC), approximately 960 infants are born with HLHS each year in the United States, i.e., one case of HLHS per 4344 live births.

The cause of HLHS is still inconclusive. Lev et al. speculated that oval foramen stenosis obstructs blood flow from the inferior vena cava to the left atrium and causes abnormal changes in intrauterine hemodynamics. Some scholars believe that hypoplasia or atresia of the left ventricular inflow and outflow tracts during the embryonic stage would lead to defects of the left ventricle and its associated aorta and mitral valve. At present, some scholars believe that mid-pregnancy fetal aortic stenosis will eventually lead to HLHS, and that arterial valvuloplasty can effectively prevent the occurrence of HLHS during the fetal period. In addition, the study also shows that HLHS is often associated with genetic abnormalities, such as NKX2.5 and GJA1 (Shay et al. 2011; Elliott et al. 2003), and with other complex genetic diseases, such as Turner and Jacobsen syndrome (Ye et al. 2010). Therefore, genetic testing should be performed in children with HLHS. At present, a large number of studies have reported that the high mortality rate of HLHS children after a staged correction is closely related to extracardiac malformations and genetic syndromes (Stasik et al. 2006). HLHS is commonly associated with other cardiac malformations including: pulmonary vein connections, coronary artery fistulas, coronary artery abnormalities, tricuspid valve defects, and vena caval abnormalities. Of patients with HLHS, 5–18% have additional extracardiac malformations, especially gastrointestinal deformities, such as esophageal atresia, duodenal atresia, malrotation of small intestine, and diaphragmatic hernia, as well as central nervous system deformities, such as agenesis corporis callosi, holoprosencephaly, and microcephaly. Death rarely occurs in fetuses with HLHS that lack a chromosomal deficiency. It should be noted that there are fundamental differences between classic HLHS and a complex deformity combined with a small left ventricle. The left ventricle in the former is small in form, far from the apex, unrelated to systemic circulation, and lacks left ventricular function; the left ventricle in the latter is also small, but is involved in systemic circulation and contains left ventricular function. Common complex malformations combined with a small left ventricle include: double outlet right ventricle (DORV) with small left ventricle, atrioventricular septal defect with small left ventricle, corrected transposition of great arteries with large ventricular septum and small left ventricle, tube-like subvalvular aortic stenosis, aortic valve stenosis, and ascending aorta and aortic arch hypoplasia with large ventricular septal defects.

References

Elliott DA, Kirk EP, Yeoh T, Chandar S, McKenzie F, Taylor P, Grossfeld P, Fatkin D, Jones O, Hayes P, Feneley M, Harvey RP. Cardiac homeobox gene NKX2-5 mutations and congenital heart disease. Associations with atrial septal defect and hypoplastic left heart syndrome. J Am Coll Cardiol. 2003;41(11):2072–6. https://doi.org/10.1016/s0735-1097(03)00420-0.

Shay A, Kirwin S, Funanage V. Hypoplastic left heart syndrome: molecular consequences of transcription factor mutations. FASEB J. 2011;25(1 Supplement):698.616.

Stasik CN, Goldberg CS, Bove EL, Devaney EJ, Ohye RG. Current outcomes and risk factors for the Norwood procedure. J Thorac Cardiovasc Surg. 2006;131(2):412–7. https://doi.org/10.1016/j.jtcvs.2005.09.030

Ye M, Coldren C, Liang X, Mattina T, Goldmuntz E, Benson DW, Ivy D, Perryman MB, Garrett-Sinha LA, Grossfeld P. Deletion of ETS-1, a gene in the Jacobsen syndrome critical region, causes ventricular septal defects and abnormal ventricular morphology in mice. Hum Mol Genet. 2010;19(4):648–56. https://doi.org/10.1093/hmg/ddp532.

Chapter 20
Surgical Treatment History

Yu Guo Weng and Bin Qiao

A series of congenital cardiovascular malformations, including hypoplasia of the left ventricular cavity, ascending aorta, and aortic arch accompanied by right heart hypertrophy was initially called left ventricular tunnel hypoplasia syndrome by Lev in 1952. In 1958, Noonan and Nadas formally named these malformations, with left ventricular obstruction and cardiac hypoplasia, accompanied by aortic and mitral valve stenosis or atresia "left ventricular hypoplasia syndrome" (Noonan and Nadas 1958).

Norwood successfully performed a two-stage corrective procedure for HLHS in 1983 (Norwood et al. 1983). The Stage I surgery was performed on an infant shortly after birth and is also known as the Stage I Norwood Surgery. Conversion of the dilated pulmonary artery main trunk into the aorta was first performed with the right ventricle functioning as the left ventricle. The atrial septum was enlarged. The divided left and right pulmonary arteries, after oversawed, were anastomosed to anonymous arteries with artificial vasculature. Thus, the systemic to pulmonary shunt, i.e., Blalock–Taussig prosthesis shunt, was established. The Stage II surgery was performed when the infant's lung circulation resistance decreased. The upper and lower venae cavae and pulmonary artery were directly connected using a half tunnel patch in the right atrium, up until the point that the final palliative single ventricle operation was accomplished. This operation was the total cavopulmonary

Y. G. Weng (✉)
German Heart Center (Berlin), Berlin, Germany
e-mail: wengyuguo@dhzb.de

B. Qiao
Cardiovascular Institute, General Hospital of Jinan Military Region, Jinan, China

Cardiac Surgery Center, Western District of Shandong Provincial Hospital, Jinan, China

B. Qiao et al. (eds.), *Surgical Atlas of Functional Single Ventricle and Hypoplastic Left Heart Syndrome*, https://doi.org/10.1007/978-981-10-8435-5_20

connection (TCPC), also known as Fontan surgery, with blood in arteries and veins separated. This two-stage corrective procedure is named the classic Norwood procedure by cardiac surgeons.

The ductus arteriosus may be closed under life-threatening conditions at any time because of high resistance of neonatal pulmonary circulation, so the first stage of the operation is necessary. The first operation is immediately followed by a total cavopulmonary connection Fontan procedure; therefore, the overall mortality rate of the classic Norwood procedure is high. A large number of clinical ultrasound examinations discovered that myocardial systolic function, the ratio of ventricular wall thickness to ventricular volume, is significantly elevated after a Fontan operation, implying that a sudden decline in the volume load of the single ventricle, which is simultaneously responsible for systemic and pulmonary circulation, leads to myocardial quality degradation and cardiac volume reduction after the total cavopulmonary connection. Changes of myocardial volume–quality relationships, which reduce myocardial systolic and diastolic function, are one of the reasons of the high early mortality rate in Fontan surgery.

Norwood was the first to stage the Fontan operation in two procedures in 1989 (Norwood 1989). Until the ventricle can adapt to this pathological circulation in respect to morphology and function by gradually reducing the single ventricular volume load, the bodily and lung circulations were completely separated. Following operation on the right atrium and completion of the pulmonary artery connection, after an incision was made in the right atrium, the inferior vena cava and pulmonary artery connection was separated with a patch in the atrium, and superior vena cava and right atrium connection was maintained normally, with the superior vena caval blood flowing directly into the pulmonary artery, and the inferior vena cava blood flowing into bodily circulation. This is done to facilitate carrying out a total cavopulmonary Fontan connection only by removing the separating patch instead of a tunnel-type patch to establish the intra-atrium lateral tunnel. The type of intermediate surgery for the Fontan surgery is called the Stage II Norwood procedure, also known as the hemi-Fontan operation.

Regarding the high mortality rate and presence of postoperative complications, a strict standard for patient selection has developed. According to years of clinical practice by cardiac surgeons all over the world and subsequent follow-up results, these surgeons discovered in the 1980s that if the classic end-to-end one-direction connection between the superior vena cava and right pulmonary artery, also known as the Glenn procedure, was modified as an end-to-side connection between the superior vena cava and left or right pulmonary artery, directing superior vena caval blood to the respective left or right pulmonary artery, the success rate of the Fontan surgery would significantly improve. To distinguish this operation from the former classic Glenn surgery, the latter is called the Glenn bi-direction shunt. The Glenn bi-direction shunt naturally became the Stage II Norwood procedure. This procedure offered the advantage of being a convenient intermediate of the final total cavopulmonary connection Fontan procedure. The final total cavopulmonary connection

Fontan surgery, whether constructed with an intra-atrial tunnel or extracardiac conduit, is called the Stage III Norwood procedure.

HLHS staged operations are palliative procedures, and the first stage of the surgery often determines the survival of sick children. As far as the surgical approach is concerned, because hypoplasia of the ascending aorta might develop to be as small as 2 mm in diameter, the size of the innominate arterial pulmonary artery shunt and how much postoperative flow it can provide will affect the prognosis. Subsequently, many surgeons have modified the Stage I Norwood procedure. There are three common improvements: (a) If the ascending aorta diameter is less than 3 mm, the small ascending aorta is cross-cut off at its junction with the aortic arch and directly end-to-side anastomosed to the neoaorta. (b) Clinical echocardiography shows diastolic "stolen blood" from the neoaorta present in the innominate arterial pulmonary artery shunt, which leads to poor postoperative coronary perfusion (Ohye et al. 2004). A right ventricular pulmonary artery shunt (Sano shunt) can avoid diastolic aortic "stolen blood," ensuring postoperative coronary perfusion, improving myocardial function, increasing cardiac output, and increasing the postoperative survival rate of the Stage I Norwood procedure. This surgical approach is such that a shunt is directly established between the right ventricular outflow tract and pulmonary artery, with a Gore-Tex artificial blood vessel diameter of approximately 5 mm (Sano shunt) (Sano et al. 2003). The disadvantage of this shunt is that it is likely to affect the postoperative ventricular function of right ventricular opening. (c) Gibbs et al. were the first to adopt a hybrid operation to treat HLHS instead of the Stage I Norwood procedure in 1992 (Gibbs et al. 1992). The advantage of this operation is avoiding the complications and potential risks of neonatal cardiopulmonary bypass and deep hypothermic circulatory arrest, while the disadvantage of this hybrid method is that the presence of a stent in the narrowed duct may cause aortic stenosis, which seriously affects perfusion in the brain and coronary arteries. Additionally, the left and right pulmonary arteries could suffer from risk of stenosis because of tissue scars. Hybrid surgery has not been extensively carried out as a replacement of the Stage I Norwood procedure; however, successful hybridization has improved the postoperative survival rate of the Stage I Norwood surgery, laying the foundation for postoperative surgical treatment.

Another alternate surgical procedure is heart transplantation. Bailey first reported in 1985 the application of a xenogeneic (baboon) heart in heart transplantation for an HLHS patient, but the recipient survived only 20 days after the operation (Bailey et al. 1985). Soon after, another cardiac transplantation with an allograft was successfully performed for an 8-day-old HLHS infant, with the donor heart stemming from a 4-day-old newborn, weighing 2.8 kg. In recent years, with pediatric technology continuously developing, cases undergoing heart transplantation have been increasing year by year; HLHS cases account for one-third to one-half of these.

The treatment of HLHS with a staged palliative surgery and heart transplantation have now been included in treatment guidelines by the Congenital Heart Association in the United States and Europe.

References

Bailey LL, Nehlsen-Cannarella SL, Concepcion W, Jolley WB. Baboon-to-human cardiac xenotransplantation in a neonate. JAMA. 1985;254(23):3321.

Gibbs JL, Rothman MT, Rees MR, Parsons JM, Blackburn ME, Ruiz CE. Stenting of the arterial duct: a new approach to palliation for pulmonary atresia. Br Heart J. 1992;67(3):240–5. https://doi.org/10.1136/hrt.67.3.240.

Noonan JA, Nadas AS. The hypoplastic left heart syndrome. Pediatr Clin North Am. 1958;5(4):1029–56. https://doi.org/10.1016/S0031-3955(16)30727-1.

Norwood WI. Hypoplastic left heart syndrome. 1989.

Norwood WI, Lang P, Hansen DD. Physiologic repair of aortic atresia–hypoplastic left heart syndrome. New Engl J Med. 1983;308(1):23–6. https://doi.org/10.1056/nejm198301063080106.

Ohye RG, Ludomirsky A, Devaney EJ, Bove EL. Comparison of right ventricle to pulmonary artery conduit and modified Blalock-Taussig shunt hemodynamics after the Norwood operation. Ann Thorac Surg. 2004;78(3):1090–3. https://doi.org/10.1016/S0003-4975(03)01386-9.

Sano S, Ishino K, Kawada M, Arai S, Kasahara S, Asai T, Masuda Z-i, Takeuchi M, Ohtsuki S-i. Right ventricle–pulmonary artery shunt in first-stage palliation of hypoplastic left heart syndrome. J Thorac Cardiovasc Surg. 2003;126(2):504–9. https://doi.org/10.1016/S0022-5223(02)73575-7.

Chapter 21
Pathological Classification

Yu Guo Weng and Bin Qiao

Pathological studies of HLHS have found that approximately 45% of HLHS cases are often associated with aortic valve atresia and mitral stenosis, 41% with aortic and mitral valve atresia, and 13% with severe aortic and mitral valve stenosis, left atrial wall thickening, and association of a patent foramen ovale or atrial septal defect. The right ventricle, pulmonary artery, and tricuspid annuli are significantly extended. The right ventricle occupies the main part of the heart apex with a sphere-like expansion about twice as large as a normal case at the same age. A patent ductus arteriosus is frequently presented in patients (PDA). The small aortic sinus still exists when aortic valve atresia is present, and the coronary artery still normally arises from the left and right sinuses. There is severe hypoplasia in the ascending aorta with a still patent lumen, with diameter ranging between 1 and 8 mm. The ascending aorta blood flows to the coronary artery with retrograde motion, acting as the only channel for coronary artery blood supply. Some cases have sinus-like hair cell vascular access from the coronary artery to the left ventricle. Eighty percent of cases are also associated with aortic arch constriction. From the view of pathology, a right ventricular single ventricle, left ventricular hypoplasia, and severe left ventricular outflow tract stenosis with a small left ventricle together constitute, along with presented intermediate forms, a disease spectrum.

Y. G. Weng (✉)
German Heart Center (Berlin), Berlin, Germany
e-mail: wengyuguo@dhzb.de

B. Qiao
Cardiovascular Institute, General Hospital of Jinan Military Region, Jinan, China

Cardiac Surgery Center, Western District of Shandong Provincial Hospital, Jinan, China

B. Qiao et al. (eds.), *Surgical Atlas of Functional Single Ventricle and Hypoplastic Left Heart Syndrome*, https://doi.org/10.1007/978-981-10-8435-5_21

Pathophysiology

The pathophysiological characteristics of HLHS are analogous to the right ventricular form of single ventricle. The anatomical right ventricle performs the pumping function of both systemic and pulmonary circulation, without almost any function in the left ventricle. Pulmonary venous blood flows into the left atrium, the right atrium through the atrial septal defect or opening foramen ovale, the right ventricle and pulmonary artery, then finally into the aorta across the ductus, so that the aorta and pulmonary artery all contain mixed blood. The carotid and coronary arteries receive mixed blood by retrograde perfusion from the aortic arch. The ratio of right heart output to the pulmonary circulation compared to the systemic circulation depends on the vascular resistance of the pulmonary and systemic circulations; a balanced body and lung perfusion can be maintained in most cases. Low pulmonary to systemic vascular resistance ratios in some cases result in excessive pulmonary blood, and although the arterial oxygen saturation can be increased, patients can still appear metabolically acidotic because of inadequate systemic blood in the marginal state. There may be a high vascular resistance ratio of pulmonary to systemic due to restrictive atrial septum among a small number of cases. Because of the lack of appropriate pulmonary blood flow, the patients might suffer bruising, hypoxemia and acidosis, with arterial PO_2 less than 20 mmHg. The patients would die if the condition deteriorates rapidly. Besides, only infants born with a patent ductus allowing pulmonary blood into the aorta can survive for several weeks to several months. HLHS infants can be successfully born, having relied on a pathological balance during the fetal stage, and should maintain this pathological balance after birth. It is a basic condition for the survival of newborns that mixed arteriovenous blood can be supplied to the whole body across the patent foramen ovale or atrial septal defect and patent ductus.

HLHS is divided into four subtypes in the clinic: (a) mitral atresia/aortic atresia (MA/AOA); (b) mitral stenosis/aortic atresia (MS/AOA); (c) mitral stenosis/aortic stenosis (MS/AOS); (d) the type of mitral atresia/aortic stenosis (MA/AOS) with a ventricular septal defect is relatively rare (Fig. 21.1).

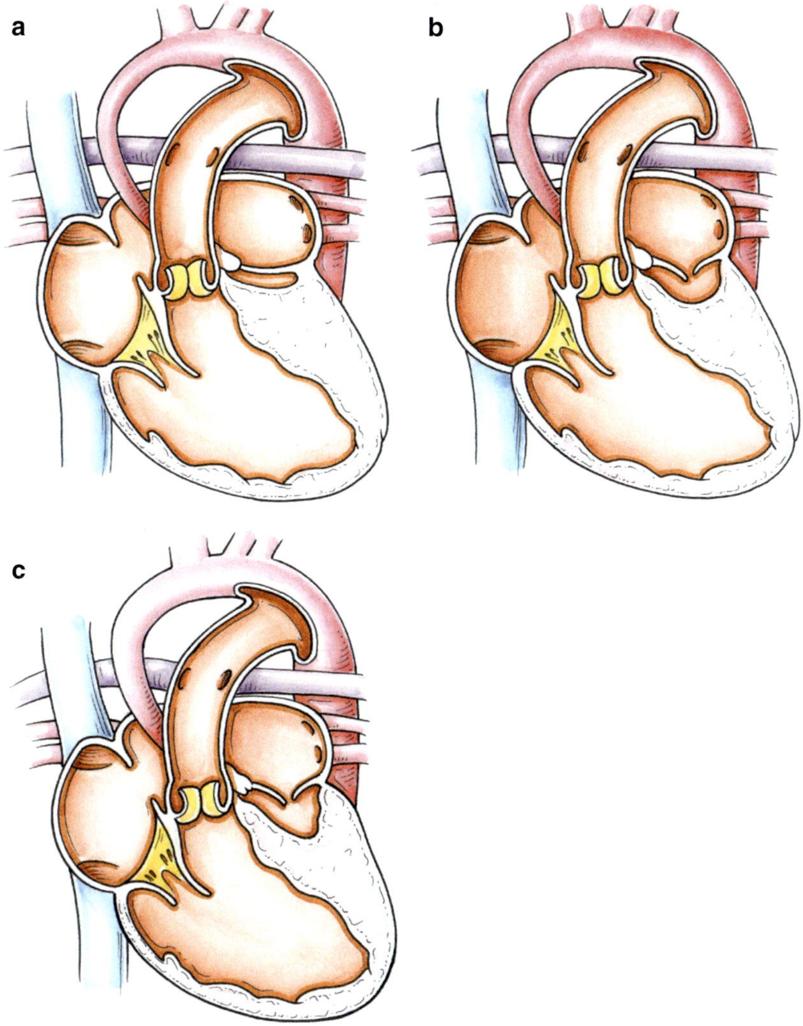

Fig. 21.1 Anatomical classification of hypoplastic left heart syndrome

Chapter 22
Indications and Contraindications

Yu Guo Weng and Bin Qiao

22.1 Surgical Indications

HLHS is a fatal disease that cannot be corrected by surgery unless a heart transplant is performed. Babies often die within 1 month after birth, and very few cases survive longer than 1 year. Once a definite diagnosis is obtained, surgery should be performed as soon as possible. It is advisable to first perform the first stage of the Norwood surgery, followed by the staged Fontan surgery. Heart transplantation is undoubtedly the best choice for treatment of HLHS. Whether just after birth or any time during the staged procedure, as long as there are no contraindications of heart transplant, the patient should be enrolled as a candidate on the heart transplant waiting list.

Contraindications of heart transplantation include:

1. The combination of other genetic diseases and incurable extracardiac deformities
2. Poor general situation, no improvement under treatment
3. Shock, liver, and kidney function impaired
4. Acute infection and pulmonary insufficiency
5. No possibility of domestic or social support after heart transplantation
6. Intellectual disability or lack of physical and mental integrity
7. Other factors unsuitable for heart transplantation

Y. G. Weng (✉)
German Heart Center (Berlin), Berlin, Germany
e-mail: wengyuguo@dhzb.de

B. Qiao
Cardiovascular Institute, General Hospital of Jinan Military Region, Jinan, China

Cardiac Surgery Center, Western District of Shandong Provincial Hospital, Jinan, China

B. Qiao et al. (eds.), *Surgical Atlas of Functional Single Ventricle and Hypoplastic Left Heart Syndrome*, https://doi.org/10.1007/978-981-10-8435-5_22

22.2 Preoperative Preparation

The success rate of the palliative surgery can be elevated by strengthened preoperative care and improvement of the general situation for a neonate with HLHS. The basic treatment is as follows: (1) Atrial septal balloon dilatation (Rashkind's procedure) should be performed as soon as possible after the patient has been transferred from the obstetrics and neonatal department to the pediatric cardiology ward; (2) Prostaglandin E should be administered intravenously with an initial dose of 10–20 ng/kg/min, and should be reduced to 5–10 ng/kg/min if the ductus arteriosus is confirmed to be patent by echocardiography; (3) Acid and alkali balance is maintained, and acidosis is handled; (4) Spontaneous breathing is advisable, instead of intubation; (5) An oxygen concentration of 20% (FiO_2) is appropriate if needed; instead of a high concentration of oxygen, oxygen saturation should be maintained at 75–80%; (6) The pressure load of the systemic circulation (using sodium nitroprusside, phentolamine, etc.) should be reduced to maintain hypotension within a normal range. (7) Stable oxygen saturation should be ensured. A blood transfusion should be appropriately performed if necessary, with an optimal hemoglobin (Hb) concentration of 140 g/L or more.

For circulatory shock or low cardiac output, the treatments are as follows: (1) Tracheal intubation ventilation should be performed to sustain a carbon dioxide partial pressure of 40–45 mmHg and an oxygen partial pressure of 40 mmHg. Too high an oxygen saturation shown by blood gas analysis likely implies excessive pulmonary blood flow, so carbon dioxide partial pressure should be elevated to a desirable level of 50 mmHg. (2) Capacity support is carried out. (3) Milrinone is preferred for support of heart function; catecholamines are less frequently employed because their pharmacological effect on the neonate is not obvious.

With the treatments mentioned above, liver and kidney function should be normal, pulmonary circulation resistance should be decreased, and the patient's general situation should be significantly improved. Only after the patient's general condition has become more stable can staged surgery be performed, and the best operative time should be chosen to be a few days later in the first week after the infant's birth.

Chapter 23
Stage I Norwood Procedure

Yu Guo Weng and Bin Qiao

For infants with HLHS, pulmonary vascular resistance is high, often due to the presence of severe pulmonary hypertension; therefore, Fontan surgery should not be performed immediately, but in stages. At present, three stages of the staged surgery are advisable: Stage I Norwood surgery (neonatal), Stage II Norwood surgery (6 months after Stage I surgery) and Stage III Norwood surgery (6 to 12 months after Hemi-Fontan surgery or bidirectional Glenn shunt). The ultimate goal of the staged reconstruction is to transition to Fontan surgery, in which the systemic and pulmonary circulations are separated, and the single ventricle sustains the entire circulation. There are three goals that need to be achieved after surgery: (1) A non-obstructive blood flow is obtained from the right ventricle to the aorta and to the coronary artery. (2) The pathway between atriums is ensured to be adequate, and pulmonary venous return is unobstructed. (3) A systemic to pulmonary shunt of appropriate size should be established to limit pulmonary blood flow and to reduce the volume load of the right ventricle.

Surgery is performed under cardiopulmonary bypass and deep hypothermia (18–20 °C of rectal temperature). The approach is through a median sternotomy. The thymus is partially excised, and the pericardium is cut open. A F8-F10 arterial cannula is inserted in the root of the pulmonary artery main trunk, and a bipolar venous cannula is placed in the inferior vena cava through the right atrium. The left and right pulmonary arteries are dissected with a sheath around them. Immediately after beginning bypass, the sheath is contracted to avoid lung perfusion. The innominate

Y. G. Weng (✉)
German Heart Center (Berlin), Berlin, Germany
e-mail: wengyuguo@dhzb.de

B. Qiao
Cardiovascular Institute, General Hospital of Jinan Military Region, Jinan, China

Cardiac Surgery Center, Western District of Shandong Provincial Hospital, Jinan, China

B. Qiao et al. (eds.), *Surgical Atlas of Functional Single Ventricle and Hypoplastic Left Heart Syndrome*, https://doi.org/10.1007/978-981-10-8435-5_23

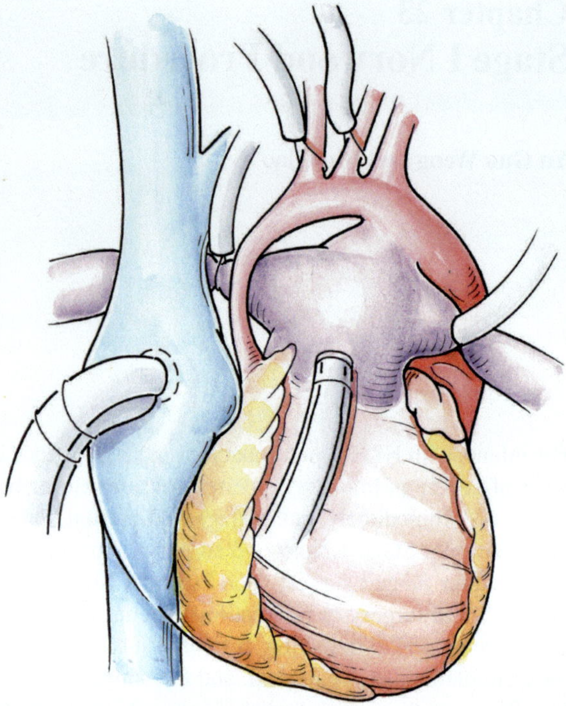

Fig. 23.1 Stage I Norwood surgery: the location of cannula

artery and left carotid artery are allowed to be dissected and surrounded with sheaths during cooling, and then cardiopulmonary bypass is started (Fig. 23.1).

The aortic arch, proximal descending aorta, and ductus are all continuously isolated and exposed. When rectal temperature drops to 18–20 °C, the sheaths around the innominate artery and the left carotid artery are tightened to avoid an air embolism in cerebral vessels. Bypass is then completely stopped. The left pulmonary artery occlusion line is removed. The arterial and venous cannulas can be pulled out after the whole-body blood has been drained into the artificial heart–lung machine. Through the right atrium cannulation purse-string suture, the atrial septum can be exposed, and all of the atrial septum should be excised. During cooling, the emptied heart appears to gradually become bradycardic flow arrests, while the heart in deep hypothermia is relaxed, soft, and pale. Cardiac activity cannot be observed with the naked eye, and the ECG is a straight line. Cardioplegia is not applied at this moment. The ductus is ligated close to its pulmonary end. The pulmonary artery is transversely divided at a position above the pulmonary valve, at the same level of the sinotubular junction of the undeveloped ascending aorta, and the pulmonary valve can be examined. The incision of the filleting ascending aorta and aortic arch is extended from the aortic sinotubular junction line, across the ascending aorta and aortic arch, and down the descending aorta to a level 1 cm below the ductus (Fig. 23.2).

Cardioplegic solutions can be inversely infused into the small ascending aorta, if needed, which can be reached through the aortic opening of the divided ductus along the aortic arch. The distal pulmonary artery incision is advisable to be oversewn by a recommended biomaterial patch, such as bovine pericardium, porcine

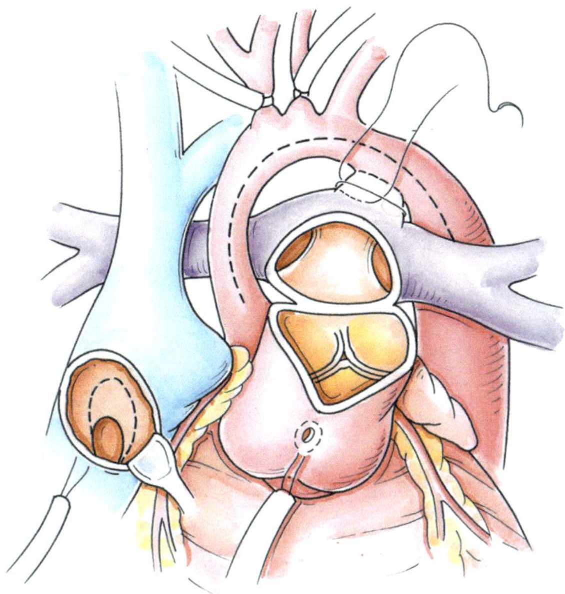

Fig. 23.2 Stage I Norwood surgery: resection of the atrium septum, transection of the pulmonary trunk, ligation of the ductus arteriosus

pericardium, allogeneic aorta, or Gore-Tex patch, using continuous Prolene between 6 and 7-0. All the ductus tissue is removed at the aortic arch. The ductus can be easily distinguished as super fragile, while normal aortic wall tissue is tough and has clear structural levels. The resulting aortotomy is extended distally as well as proximally along the undersurface of the arch and the medial edge of the ascending aorta to a level about 5 mm above the aortic valve, equivalent to the aortic sinotubular junction line. Care should be taken not to extend too far to avoid sinotubular junction stenosis with poor coronary perfusion through possible excessive tissue traction when the aorta is repaired (Fig. 23.3).

An allogeneic patch is shaped for enlargement of the aorta and its arch, referring to what Fig. 23.4 illustrates. First, suturing of the back wall is performed using 6-0 continuous Prolene with a double needle suture, starting from the descending aortic incision in the arch. To facilitate the operation, the pulmonary-end anastomosis of the systemic and pulmonary prosthesis shunt (Blalock–Taussig prosthesis shunt) is first treated using 7-0 sutures with a fine needle. The shunt can be made using 3 or 3.5 mm Gore-Tex artificial blood vessels with rings, with their diameter depending on the size of the neonate. After completion, the artificial blood vessels are stretched to the innominate artery under the aorta.

Figure 23.5 shows the preferred reshaping and formation of the ascending aorta and arch. After continuous suturing of the posterior and anterior walls is completed, each end of continuous sutures is pierced the aorta outside through the anterior or posterior wall and sinotubular junction at ascending aorta, then tightened with knots respectively. Care should be taken that the connection between the patch and the anterior and posterior walls of the ascending aorta is rectangular; otherwise sinotubular junction stenosis might occur because of improper stitching, pulling, or twisting to the proximal end of the ascending aorta.

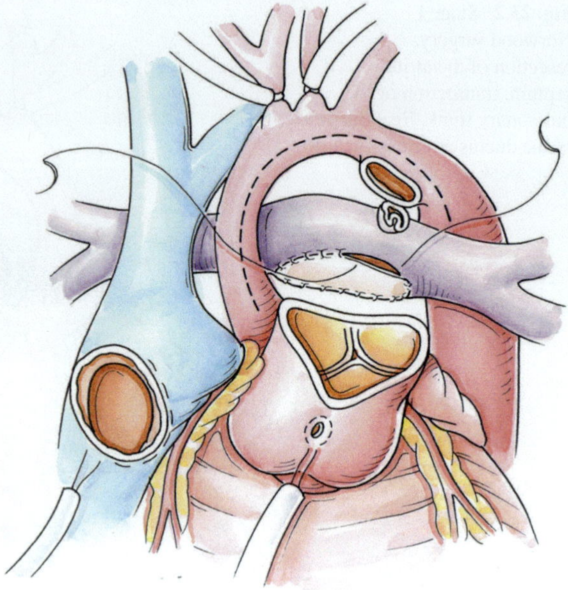

Fig. 23.3 Stage I Norwood surgery: incision closing of distal pulmonary artery, removal of ductus arteriosus tissue

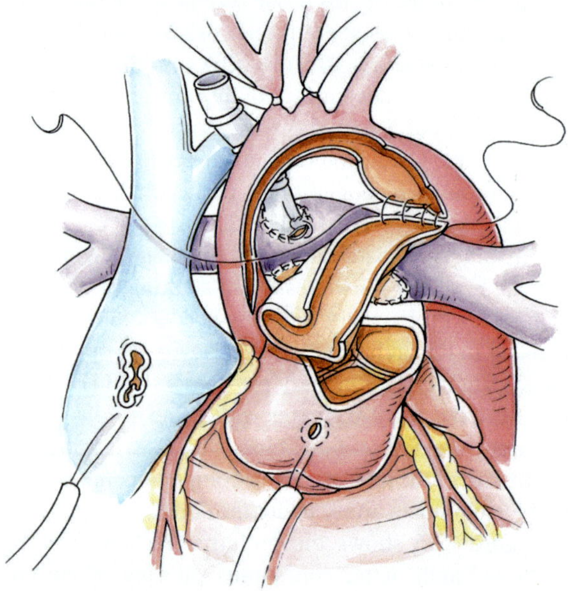

Fig. 23.4 Stage I Norwood surgery: incision and expansion of the ascending aorta and its arch, anastomosing the end of bypass vessel to the pulmonary artery

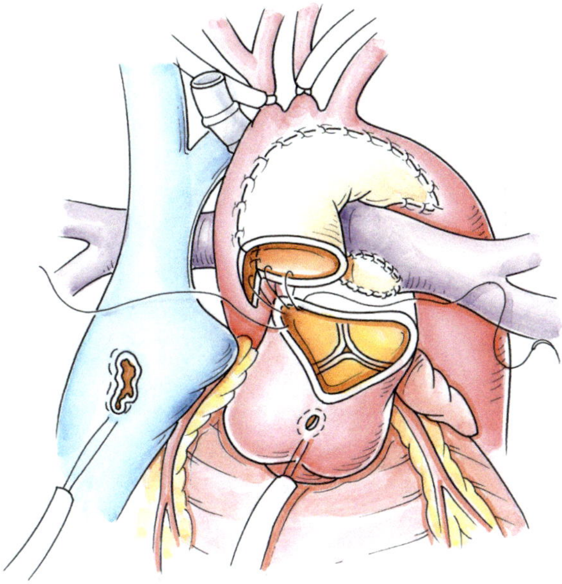

Fig. 23.5 Stage I Norwood surgery: ascending aorta and its arch formation

The neoaorta anastomosis has been completed, and arterial and venous cannulas are placed at the original intubation site. Air venting of the brain and the heart are performed. (Before bypass recovery, the aorta is filled with blood in a head-down position for ascending aorta venting; after releasing the rubber sleeve around the innominate artery and the left carotid artery, brain venting is performed.) Following heart venting, cardiopulmonary bypass is begun again, and gradually rewarming should last at least 45 min. During rewarming, the proximal anastomosis of the Blalock–Taussig prosthesis to the innominate artery can be performed. After completion of the artificial vascular shunts, rewarming is continued with temporary clamping of the Gore-Tex shunt. When nasopharyngeal temperature has reached 25~30 °C, calcium concentration should be monitored and immediately corrected if lower than normal. Once rewarming is complete, the pump is stopped, and the bodily pulmonary shunt is opened. Ultrafiltration is performed prior to neutralization with heparin to discharge excessive water in the body as soon as possible. Bypass pipelines are removed. A monitoring catheter is placed in the right atrium, myocardial leads are set in the right atrium and right ventricle for later pacing use, and the chest is routinely closed (Fig. 23.6).

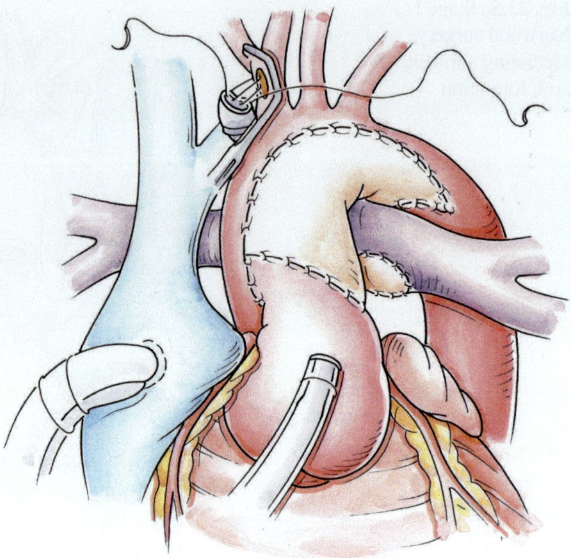

Fig. 23.6 Stage I Norwood surgery: anastomosing the end of bypass vessel to innominate artery

Chapter 24
Stage I Modified Norwood Procedure

Yu Guo Weng and Bin Qiao

Two approaches can be taken in the Stage I modified Norwood procedure: (1) For an extremely hyperplastic ascending aorta, its diameter is only 2-3mm, that is, much smaller than the aortic sinus. The classic Norwood ascending aorta formation method is likely to cause sinotubular junction stenosis, resulting in poor coronary artery perfusion. Using the modified approach, the ascending aorta, which has developed extremely poorly, is transversely divided at its junction with the aortic arch and directly end-to-side anastomosed to the neoaorta. (2) The innominate to pulmonary arterial shunt (Blalock-Taussig shunt) is replaced by a right ventricle to pulmonary arterial shunt (Sano Shunt). It offers the advantage of avoiding diastolic "stolen blood" from the ascending aorta of the Blalock-Taussig shunt to ensure that the new ascending aorta fills in diastole, which is conducive to coronary perfusion and cardiac function recovery. The disadvantage of this shunt is that a right ventricular incision may damage ventricular contractile function. A Gore-Tex artificial blood vessel with a diameter of about 5-6mm may be selected to connect the pulmonary artery and the right ventricle; other artificial materials or allogeneic blood vessels are also available and can be placed on either side of the neoaorta.

Cardiopulmonary bypass and intubation techniques are the same as the Stage I classic Norwood procedure. All cannulas are removed after circulatory arrest, the right atrium is exposed through the vein intubation opening, and all redundant atrial septal tissue is removed. The ascending aorta is then divided at its junction with the aortic arch. All redundant ductus tissue on the aorta and pulmonary artery is excised.

Y. G. Weng (✉)
German Heart Center (Berlin), Berlin, Germany
e-mail: wengyuguo@dhzb.de

B. Qiao
Cardiovascular Institute, General Hospital of Jinan Military Region, Jinan, China

Cardiac Surgery Center, Western District of Shandong Provincial Hospital, Jinan, China

B. Qiao et al. (eds.), *Surgical Atlas of Functional Single Ventricle and Hypoplastic Left Heart Syndrome*, https://doi.org/10.1007/978-981-10-8435-5_24

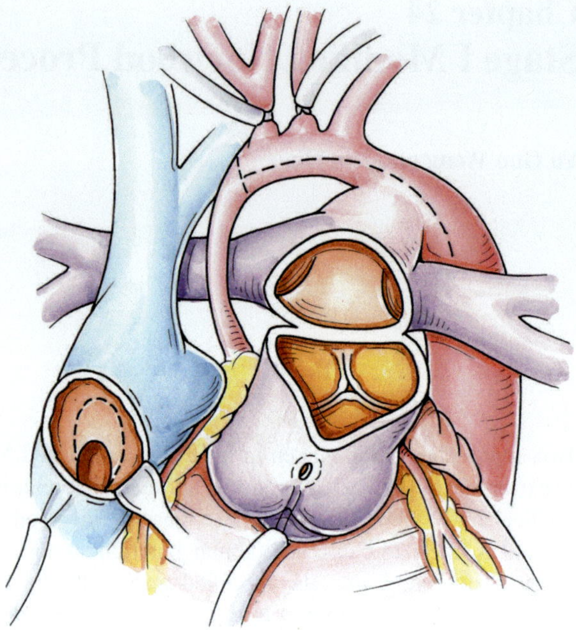

Fig. 24.1 Stage I modified Norwood procedure: resection of the atrium septum, transection of the ascending aorta and pulmonary trunk

The poorly developed aortic arch is filleted along the dotted line to the normal descending aorta. The pulmonary artery main trunk is transected at the point of left and right pulmonary artery bifurcation (Fig. 24.1).

The allogeneic aortic homograft, with or without valves, is prepared. The aortic arch and pulmonary artery trunk are connected using the ascending aortic segment of the aortic homograft, and a new ascending aorta is thus formed. A proximal end anastomosis is performed, beginning with the back wall, with end-to-end continuous 6-0 Prolene. The shaping of the two anastomoses of the neoaorta is relatively simpler than in the classic Norwood procedure (Fig. 24.2).

After the proximal anastomosis, the homograft is cut to length according to the distance from the proximal anastomosis to the arch, and the distal anastomosis of the neoaorta is performed. The anastomosis method is as same as the proximal anastomosis; however, the proximal opening of the hyperplastic arch should be included (Fig. 24.3).

Duct tissue should be excised normal to the pulmonary artery wall. Figure 24.4 shows the complete opening of the pulmonary artery tissue, and that the incision edges are smooth and sharp. Because so much ductus tissue is removed, closure of continuous sutures may cause pulmonary artery stenosis. With such a large ductus incision, it is appropriate to close it with a Gore-Tex or biological patch. Its cardiac-end opening can be closed with continuous sutures as more tissue from the pulmonary artery main trunk was left. A Gore-Tex vessel (5–6 mm in diameter) for the systemic-to-pulmonary artery shunt is preplaced at an appropriate location on the left pulmonary artery. Figure 24.4 shows an artificial vessel with rings.

The hyperplastic small ascending aorta is end-to-side anastomosed to the neoaorta using 7-0 Prolene sutures. Since the ascending aorta is so slim and is the only

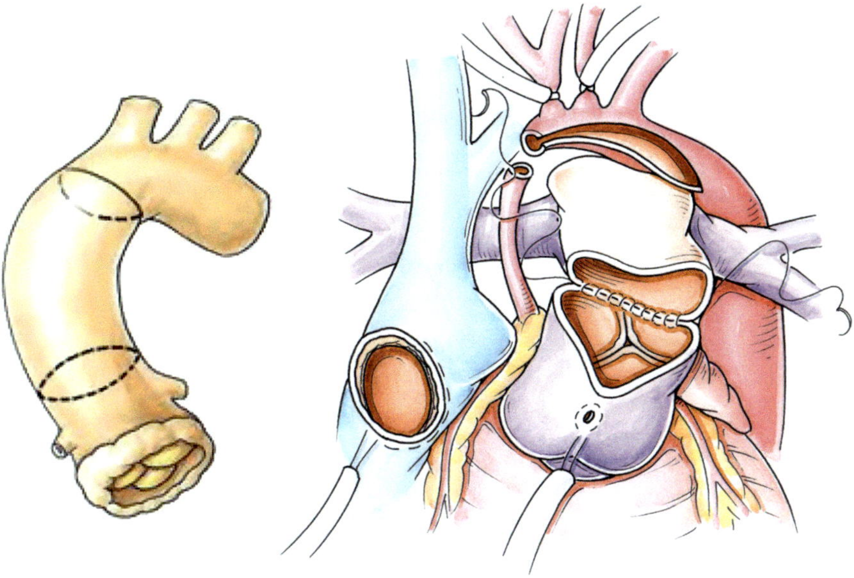

Fig. 24.2 Stage I modified Norwood procedure: connection between pulmonary artery and aortic arch with allogeneic aortic graft

Fig. 24.3 Stage I modified Norwood procedure: distal anastomosis at the new aortic

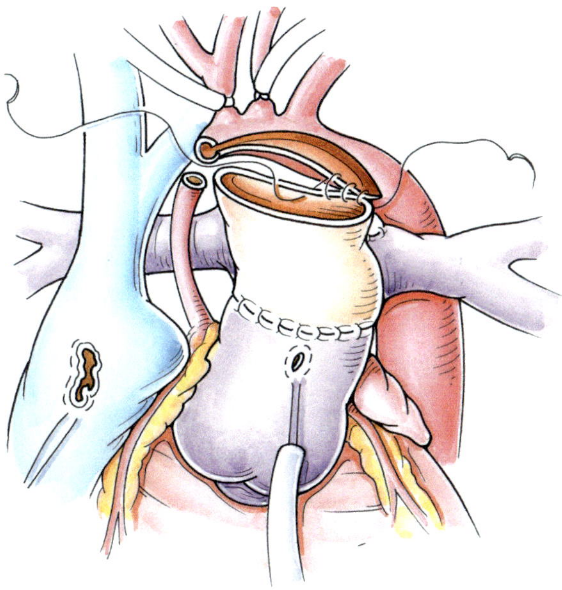

perfusion port for the coronary artery, it is very important to precisely select the location of the anastomosis in order to avoid distortion after filling, tension, or angled bending resulting from improper length. Therefore, it is advisable to anteriorly locate the anastomosis on the lateral side of the allograft. After air venting, the

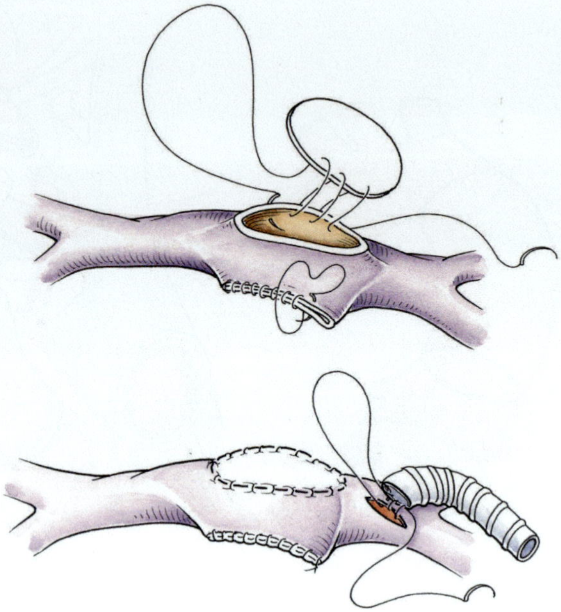

Fig. 24.4 Stage I modified Norwood procedure: resection of the ductus arteriosus, closing pulmonary artery with patch, indwelling artificial blood vessel for systemic-to-pulmonary artery shunt

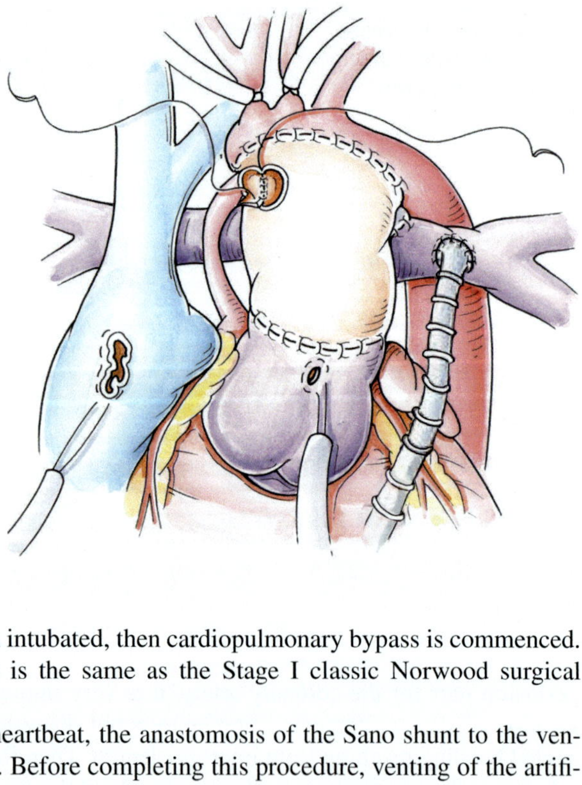

Fig. 24.5 Stage I modified Norwood procedure: anastomosing the fine ascending aorta with new ascending aorta

veins and arteries are again intubated, then cardiopulmonary bypass is commenced. The rewarming procedure is the same as the Stage I classic Norwood surgical method (Fig. 24.5).

Before recovering the heartbeat, the anastomosis of the Sano shunt to the ventricle should be performed. Before completing this procedure, venting of the artifi-

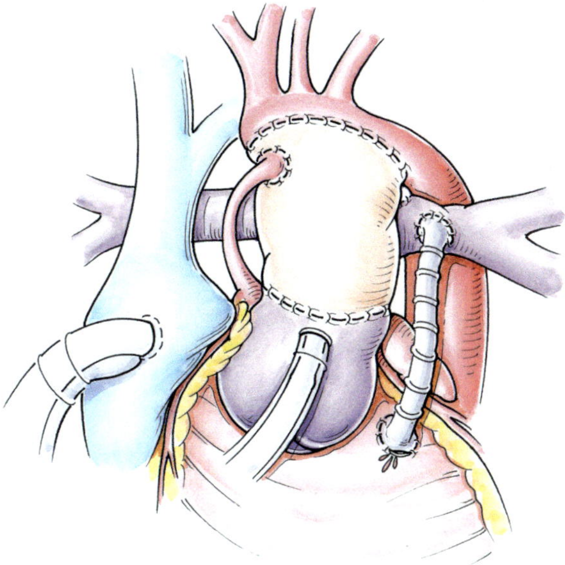

Fig. 24.6 Stage I modified Norwood procedure: to complete anastomosis of ventricular end of systemic-to-pulmonary artery shunt

cial blood vessels should be first performed. When knots are tied, the artificial blood vessel is still clamped closed. The Sano shunt needs to be gradually opened while CPB flow is reduced. When CPB has completely ceased, the shunt should be fully open (Fig. 24.6).

Chapter 25
Classic Single Fontan Procedure

Yu Guo Weng and Bin Qiao

This operation is still performed under cardiopulmonary bypass. The surgery will last a long time, being a reoperation, so moderate hypothermia (28–32 °C) is necessary. Cannulas are placed in the ascending aorta, the superior vena cava close to the innominate vein, and the inferior vena cava near the diaphragm. The systemic-to-pulmonary shunt pipeline is dissected and sewn closed once cardiopulmonary bypass has begun. After blocking the ascending aorta, HTK cardioplegia solution is perfused at a rate of 150–200 mL (40–50 mL/kg) per 8 minutes. The dashed line shows the pulmonary artery and right atrial incision which will act as the inlets from the superior and inferior venae cavae to the pulmonary artery after the connection is complete. The right atrial incision should be kept away from the superior crest at the right atrium entrance of the superior vena cava to avoid impairing the sinoatrial node (Fig. 25.1).

The posterior wall of the atrial-pulmonary connection is sutured first. The lower edge of the right pulmonary artery incision is anastomosed to the right superior vena cava—right atrial incision, and then two ends of the suture are knotted. (Fig. 25.2).

The anterior wall of the right atrium is incised along the longitudinal axis of the inferior and superior venae cavae, with the incision extending upwards and downwards to the right atrial junction of the inferior and superior venae cavae. A Gore-Tex patch is employed, shaped as a semi-tunnel, and cut to length according to the distance between the inferior and superior vena caval openings. In the middle of the

Y. G. Weng (✉)
German Heart Center (Berlin), Berlin, Germany
e-mail: wengyuguo@dhzb.de

B. Qiao
Cardiovascular Institute, General Hospital of Jinan Military Region, Jinan, China

Cardiac Surgery Center, Western District of Shandong Provincial Hospital, Jinan, China

B. Qiao et al. (eds.), *Surgical Atlas of Functional Single Ventricle and Hypoplastic Left Heart Syndrome*, https://doi.org/10.1007/978-981-10-8435-5_25

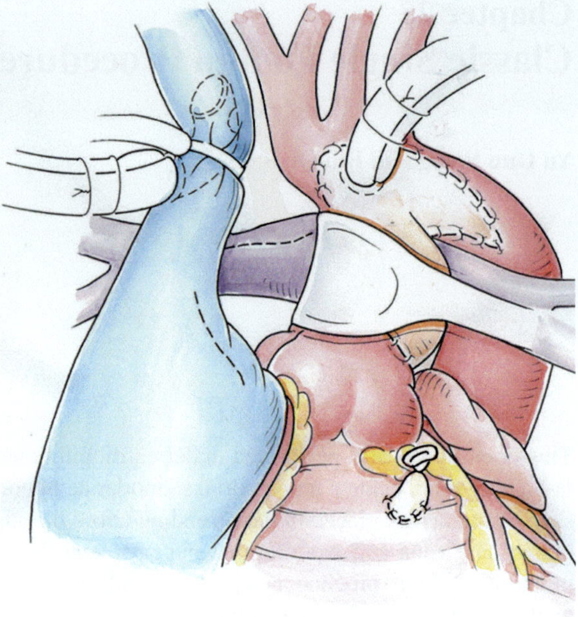

Fig. 25.1 Classic single Fontan surgery: suturing artificial blood vessel for systemic-to-pulmonary artery shunt, making incision of pulmonary artery and right atrium

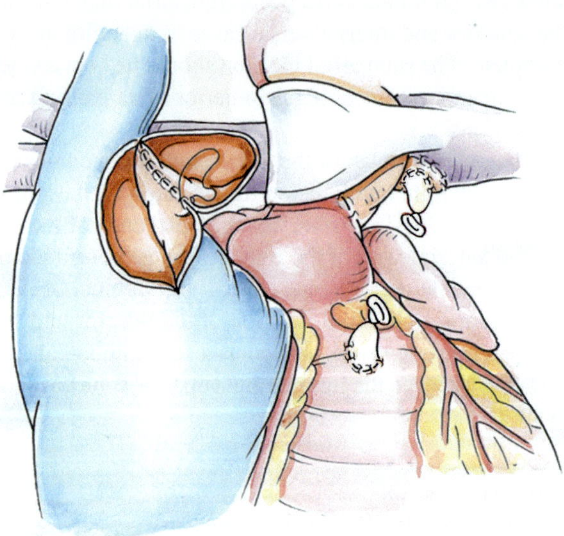

Fig. 25.2 Classic single Fontan surgery: suturing the posterior wall of anastomosis between the right atrium and pulmonary artery

patch, a 4 mm hole is opened to shunt excessive venous blood flow. An intracardiac tunnel is established using this patch to lead the inferior vena caval blood into the pulmonary artery. The residual edge of the atrial septum and left atrial opening of four pulmonary veins can be seen at the edge of the posterior wall of the tunnel. The anastomosis of the inferior end of the tunnel to the inferior vena cava is located in the right atrium and should be sufficiently large. Its superior end directly connects the right atrium to the pulmonary artery anastomosis (Fig. 25.3).

The right atrial incision is closed with continuous suturing (Fig. 25.4).

The anastomosis of right atrium to the pulmonary artery is closed with a triangular Gore-Tex patch (Fig. 25.5).

Recovery of cardiopulmonary bypass is begun, with temperature rewarming to 37 °C. A pressure catheter is placed in the right atrium and is used for postoperative pressure monitoring. Cardiopulmonary bypass is stopped, and the chest is closed routinely. In a successful Fontan operation, the inferior and superior venae cavae are directly connected to the pulmonary artery through the intracardiac tunnel. Oxygenated blood flows into the right ventricle through the defective atrial septum, tricuspid valve, and then into systemic circulation through the neoaorta (Fig. 25.6).

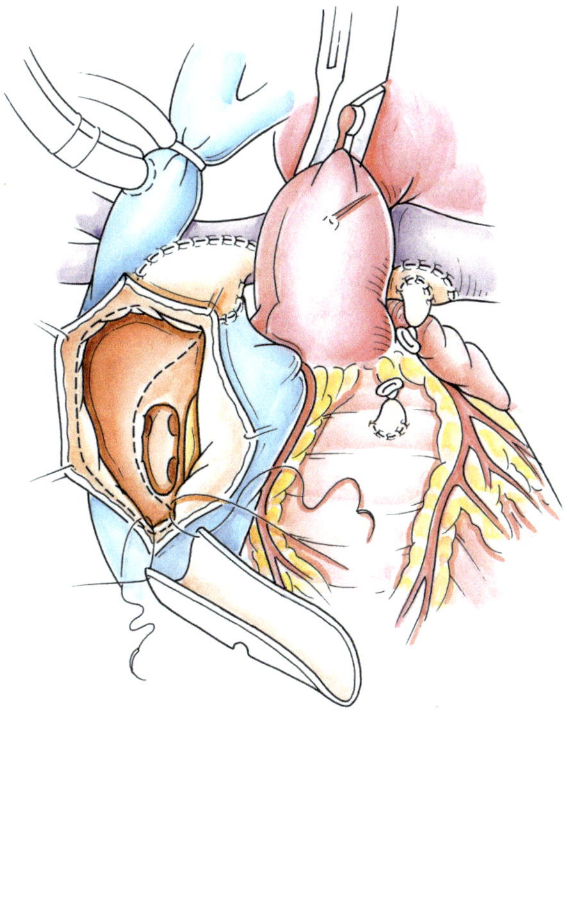

Fig. 25.3 Classic single Fontan surgery: suturing tunnel patch with a hole in right atrium

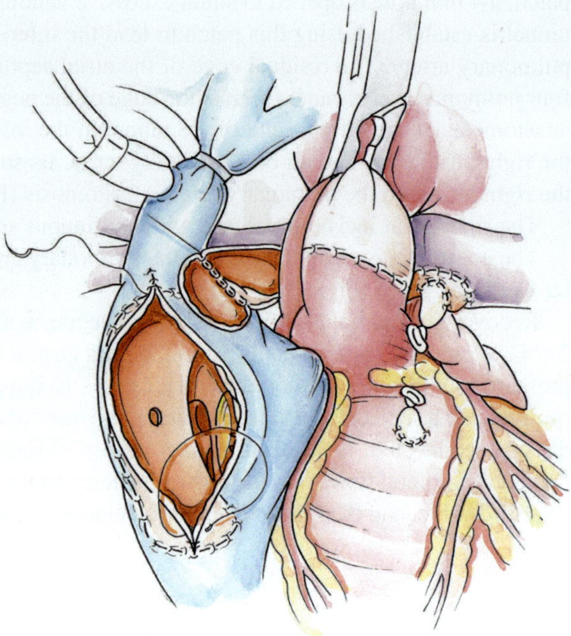

Fig. 25.4 Classic single Fontan surgery: suturing the right atrium incision

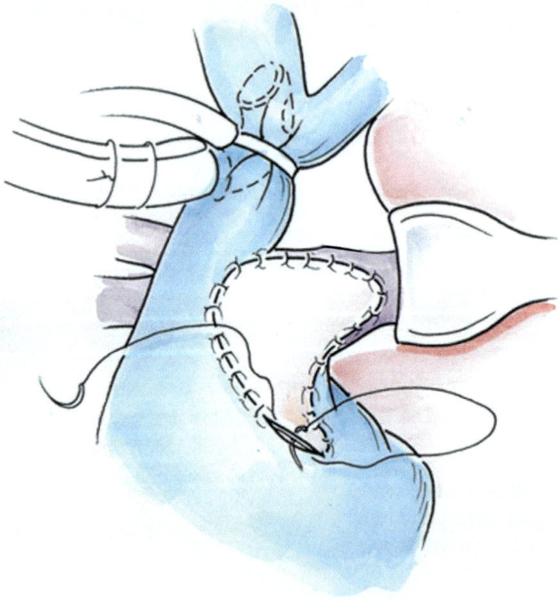

Fig. 25.5 Classic single Fontan surgery: patching the anterior wall of the anastomosis of right atrium and pulmonary artery

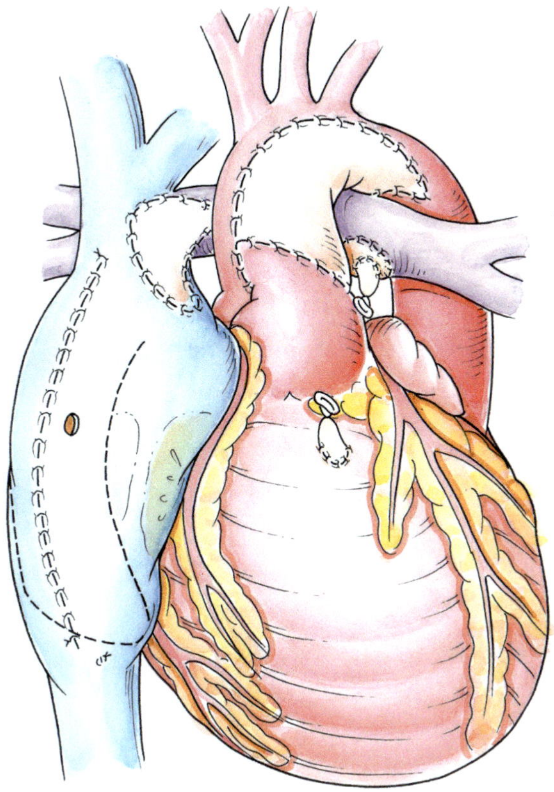

Fig. 25.6 Classic single Fontan surgery: postoperative schematic

Chapter 26
Stage II Norwood Procedure: Hemi-Fontan Surgery

Yu Guo Weng and Bin Qiao

Norwood initially adopted the single Fontan procedure with a total cavopulmonary connection in the surgical treatment of hypoplastic left heart syndrome. Whether the surgical mortality or long-term mortality rates are very high. a large number of clinical experiments regarding the cavopulmonary connection for functional single ventricle have found that myocardial systolic function and the ratio of ventricular wall thickness to ventricular volume significantly increase after Fontan surgery. It might be deduced that, after implementation of a total cavopulmonary connection, the suddenly declined volume load of the single ventricle, which simultaneously sustains the systemic and pulmonary circulations, may contribute to myocardial quality degradation and cardiac volume reduction. Changes of myocardial volume-quality relationships could reduce myocardial systolic and diastolic function and might be the reason for the high overall mortality rate of one-time total cavopulmonary connections after the first stage of treatment for hypoplastic left heart syndrome.

A connection between the right pulmonary artery and the right atrium is generally adopted in the hemi-Fontan surgery. The incision method is analogous to the single Fontan surgery (Fig. 26.1).

In the classic Norwood hemi-Fontan surgery, only one patch is applied, not only to complete the cavopulmonary anastomosis, but also to separate the blood in the inferior vena cava from that in pulmonary artery (see Figs. 14.1, 14.2, 14.3, and 14.4). In the modified hemi-Fontan operation, the right pulmonary artery is first

Y. G. Weng (✉)
German Heart Center (Berlin), Berlin, Germany
e-mail: wengyuguo@dhzb.de

B. Qiao
Cardiovascular Institute, General Hospital of Jinan Military Region, Jinan, China

Cardiac Surgery Center, Western District of Shandong Provincial Hospital, Jinan, China

B. Qiao et al. (eds.), *Surgical Atlas of Functional Single Ventricle and Hypoplastic Left Heart Syndrome*, https://doi.org/10.1007/978-981-10-8435-5_26

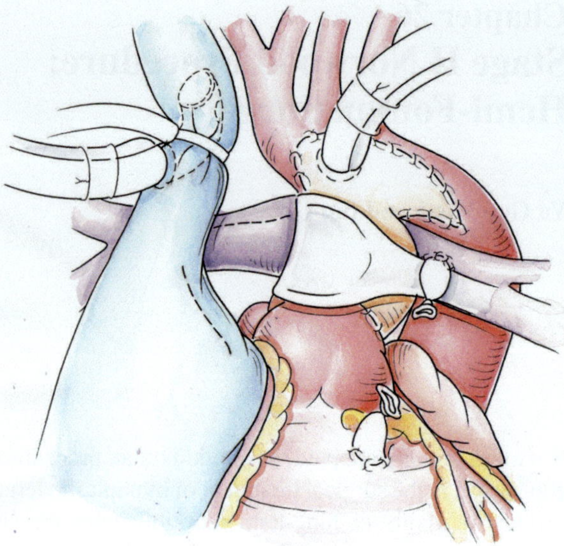

Fig. 26.1 Hemi-Fontan surgery: suturing artificial blood vessel for systemic-to-pulmonary artery shunt, making incision of pulmonary artery and right atrium

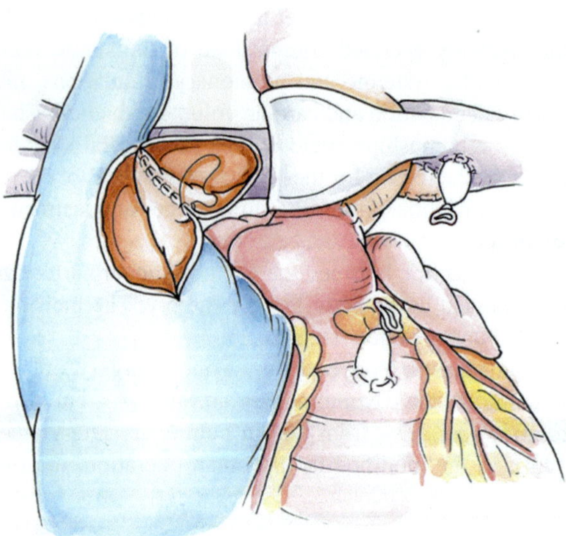

Fig. 26.2 Hemi-Fontan surgery: suturing the posterior wall of anastomosis of the right atrium to pulmonary artery

sutured to the right atrial rear wall with continuous sutures, and then the two suture ends are tightened (Fig. 26.2).

Blood flow from the superior vena cava is blocked from entering the right atrium and diverted into the pulmonary artery by placing a round Gore-Tex patch at the level of the inferior edge of the right atrial incision. The anastomosis of the right atrium to the pulmonary artery is also sewn closed with a Gore-Tex patch (Fig. 26.3).

After the hemi-Fontan operation, superior vena caval blood flows directly into pulmonary artery circulation, and inferior vena caval blood flows through the tricuspid

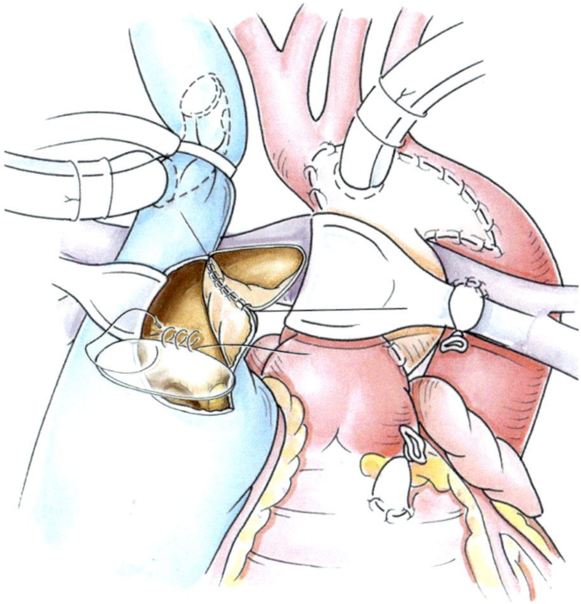

Fig. 26.3 Hemi-Fontan surgery: closing with patch the blood flow from superior vena cava into the right atrium, patching the anterior wall of the anastomosis of right atrium and pulmonary artery

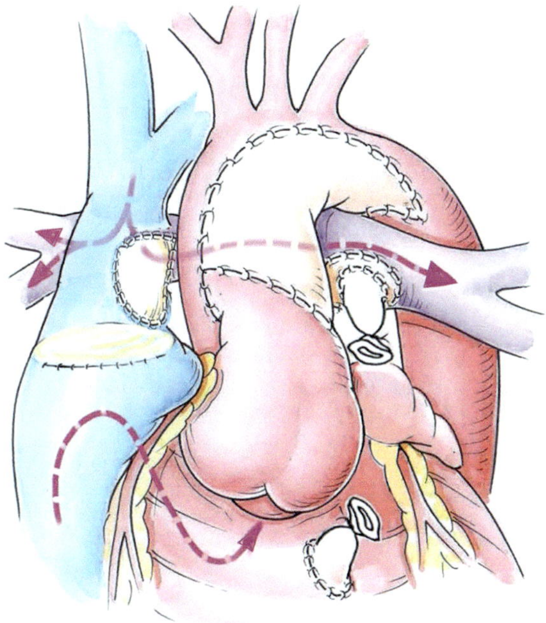

Fig. 26.4 Hemi-Fontan surgery: postoperative intracardiac flow pattern

valve into systemic circulation. The reason for which the procedure is called hemi-Fontan surgery is that the total cavopulmonary connection can be accomplished with the condition that the patch at the inlet of the superior vena cava can be removed, and a half-tunnel patch can then be added in the right atrium (Fig. 26.4).

Chapter 27
Stage II Norwood Procedure: Bidirectional Glenn Shunt

Yu Guo Weng and Bin Qiao

In the classic Glenn shunt, the divided superior vena cava is end-to-end anastomosed to the divided right pulmonary artery, with superior vena caval blood flow only to the right pulmonary artery in one direction. However, in the bidirectional Glenn shunt, the divided superior vena cava is directly anastomosed to the right pulmonary artery, with superior vena caval blood flowing into both the right and left pulmonary arteries.

After the Stage I Norwood operation, the pulmonary circulation mainly receives mixed blood through the Sano shunt. Here, the shunt is an artificial blood vessel without a reinforcement ring. The dashed line shows the division site of the superior vena cava, as close as it should be to the middle of the right pulmonary artery horizontal axis to avoid tension resulting from the side-to-end anastomosis of the inferior and superior venae cavae to the pulmonary artery. The postoperative pathophysiology of hypoplastic left heart syndrome after the first stage Norwood operation is different from functional single ventricle; the surgical methods of the second stage Glenn bidirectional shunt also vary. After endotracheal intubation and general anesthesia, with the supply of pure oxygen, the superior vena cava is blocked. In patients with excellent oxygen saturation, the bidirectional Glenn shunt surgery can be performed without cardiopulmonary bypass (Fig. 27.1).

The surgery can also be performed under normothermic bypass with the heart beating. The ascending aorta and inferior and superior venae cavae are cannulated,

Y. G. Weng (✉)
German Heart Center (Berlin), Berlin, Germany
e-mail: wengyuguo@dhzb.de

B. Qiao
Cardiovascular Institute, General Hospital of Jinan Military Region, Jinan, China

Cardiac Surgery Center, Western District of Shandong Provincial Hospital, Jinan, China

B. Qiao et al. (eds.), *Surgical Atlas of Functional Single Ventricle and Hypoplastic Left Heart Syndrome*, https://doi.org/10.1007/978-981-10-8435-5_27

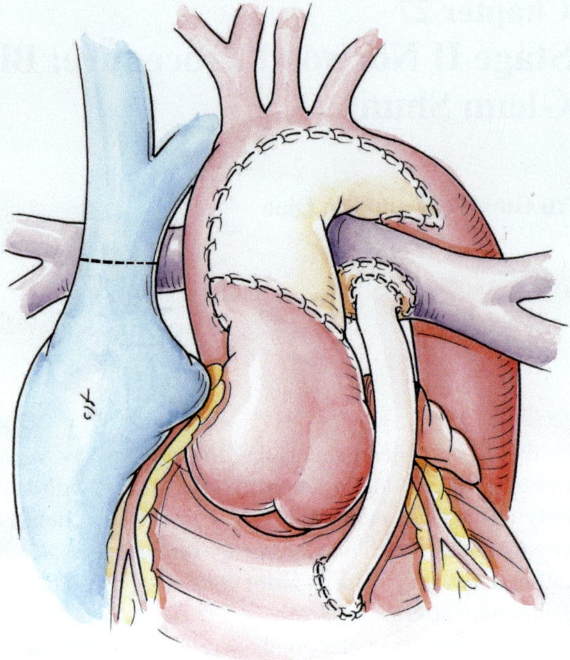

Fig. 27.1 Bidirectional Glenn shunt: the transection site of superior vena cava indicated with dashed line

and the cross-clamp at the ascending aorta is not applied. The systemic-to-pulmonary artery shunt, which is made of other materials here, is divided after CPB has begun. The right pulmonary artery incision is near the proximal portion of the pulmonary artery. To place the extracardiac conduit on the right pulmonary artery during a subsequent total Fontan operation, the right pulmonary artery is proximally or distally anastomosed to the superior vena cava (Fig. 27.2).

The tourniquet around the superior vena cava is tightened. The superior vena cava is transversely divided away from the sinoatrial node, and its proximal incision is closed with continuous sutures. The free end of the superior vena cava is anastomosed to the pulmonary artery with continuous 6-0 Prolene sutures (Fig. 27.3).

Figure 27.4 indicates the accomplished cavopulmonary anastomosis. The superior vena caval blood flows to the left and right pulmonary arteries. This is the bidirectional Glenn shunt of the Stage II Norwood procedure.

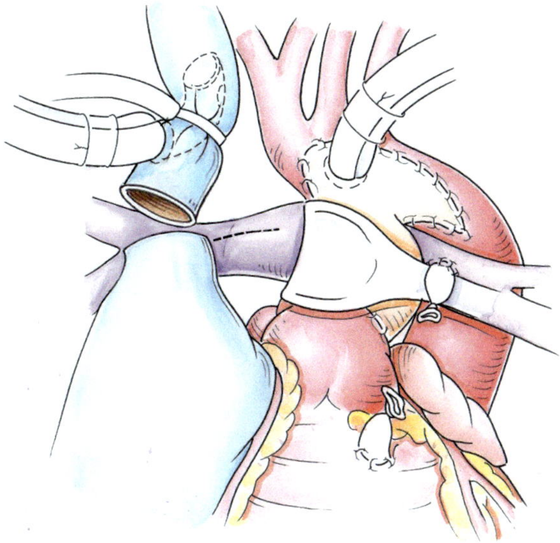

Fig. 27.2 Bidirectional Glenn shunt: cutting artificial blood vessel for systemic-to-pulmonary shunt, making the incision of right pulmonary artery

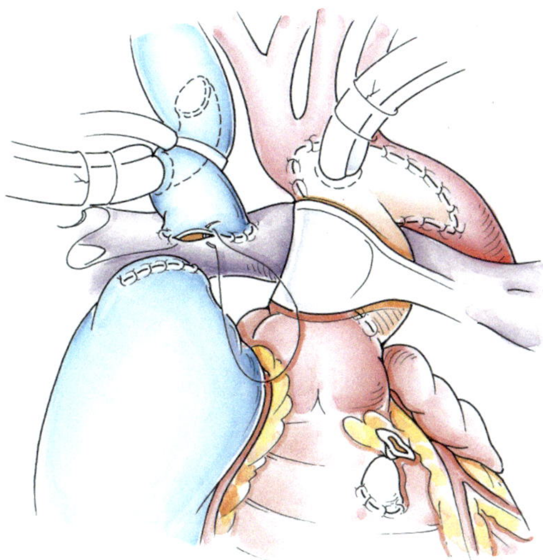

Fig. 27.3 Bidirectional Glenn shunt: the transection of superior vena cava, closing its proximal end, anastomosing its distal end with right pulmonary artery

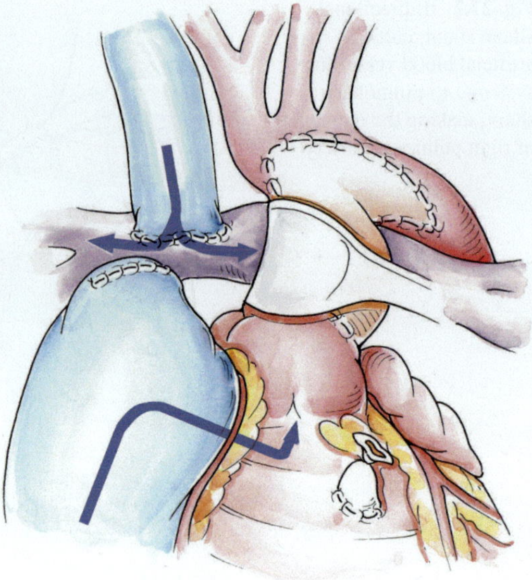

Fig. 27.4 Bidirectional Glenn shunt: postoperative intracardiac blood flow direction

Chapter 28
Stage III Norwood Surgery: Fontan Operation

Yu Guo Weng and Bin Qiao

The establishment of a lateral tunnel along the free right atrial wall can avoid resulting pulmonary venous obstructions at the entrance of the atrium because of right atrial tunnel dilatation; moreover, it can reduce supraventricular arrhythmia and atrial natriuretic peptide secretion because of the elevated right atrial pressure. Figure 28.1 shows the heart's postoperative connections after Stages I and II of the Norwood operation. The operation should be performed under cardiopulmonary bypass, at a normal temperature with the heart beating; ascending aorta occlusion is not needed. The ascending aorta and superior and inferior vena cava are cannulated. The artificial vessel used for the Sano shunt between the right ventricular outflow tract and pulmonary artery is ligated immediately after starting bypass.

After the full-flow bypass is steady, tourniquets around the inferior and superior venae cavae are tightened. First, the inferior vena cava is divided from the right atrium (with a portion of the right atrial wall to increase anastomotic diameter), and the stump of the right atrium is closed with continuous suturing. The superior end of the extracardiac conduit is continuously anastomosed to the inferior surface of the right pulmonary artery. The extracardiac conduit can be made of homograft or artificial materials. Allografts are difficult to obtain, so a Gore-Tex artificial vascular graft with loops is often selected, and its diameter should depend on the patient's weight and the size of the inferior vena cava. Regardless of the conduit's material, it cannot grow alongside an infant. To reduce the potential burden of systemic venous circulation, a fenestration is frequently applied between the extracardiac

Y. G. Weng (✉)
German Heart Center (Berlin), Berlin, Germany
e-mail: wengyuguo@dhzb.de

B. Qiao
Cardiovascular Institute, General Hospital of Jinan Military Region, Jinan, China

Cardiac Surgery Center, Western District of Shandong Provincial Hospital, Jinan, China

B. Qiao et al. (eds.), *Surgical Atlas of Functional Single Ventricle and Hypoplastic Left Heart Syndrome*, https://doi.org/10.1007/978-981-10-8435-5_28

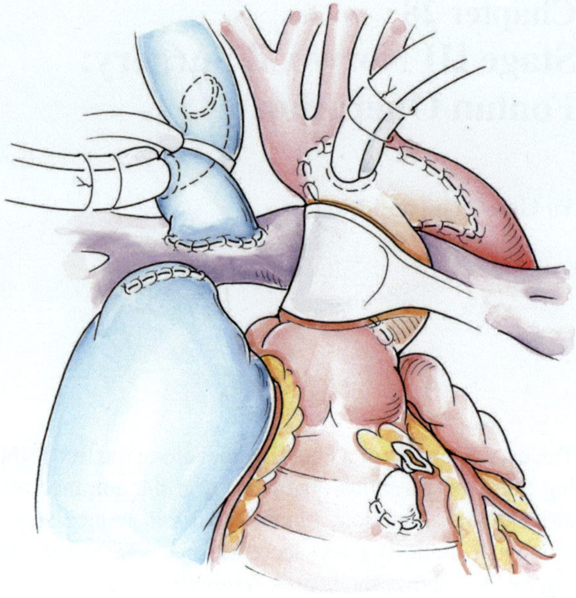

Fig. 28.1 Total cavopulmonary connection with extracardiac conduit: cutting off Sano shunt vessel

tunnel and the bypassed right atrium, and it can be occluded by an intervention technique when not required (Fig. 28.2).

Figure 28.3 shows the postoperative connection after the Stage I Norwood and hemi-Fontan operations. The right atrium and pulmonary artery are already connected; however, the superior vena cava is separated from the right atrium by a right atrium patch, and blood from the superior vena cava only flows directly into the left and right pulmonary arteries.

The whole procedure should be carried out inside the heart, so normothermic or moderate hypothermia bypass is needed with myocardial protection under cardiac arrest. The Sano shunt is ligated immediately after commencing bypass. Cardioplegia is infused after the ascending aorta has been blocked. The right atrium is cut along the longitudinal axis of the inferior and superior venae cavae, and the pre-set patch in the superior right atrium is removed; at this point, through the superior vena caval inlet, a large atrial septal defect and left and right pulmonary venous openings in the left atrium can be exposed (Fig. 28.4).

A half-tunnel patch is obtained after an artificial vascular graft that is 10 mm in diameter is longitudinally filleted (a 4 mm in diameter hole in the middle of patch is used to alleviate the circulating load of the vena cava). The resulting patch is shaped to length to correspond to the entrance of the inferior and superior venae cavae. After being trimmed, the edge of the patch to the outer wall of the atrium should be slightly shorter than that to the inner wall. The suturing procedure is begun from the inferior vena caval inlet of the right atrium. The dashed line indicates the suturing path of the intracardiac half tunnel. The back wall is sutured upward along the edge

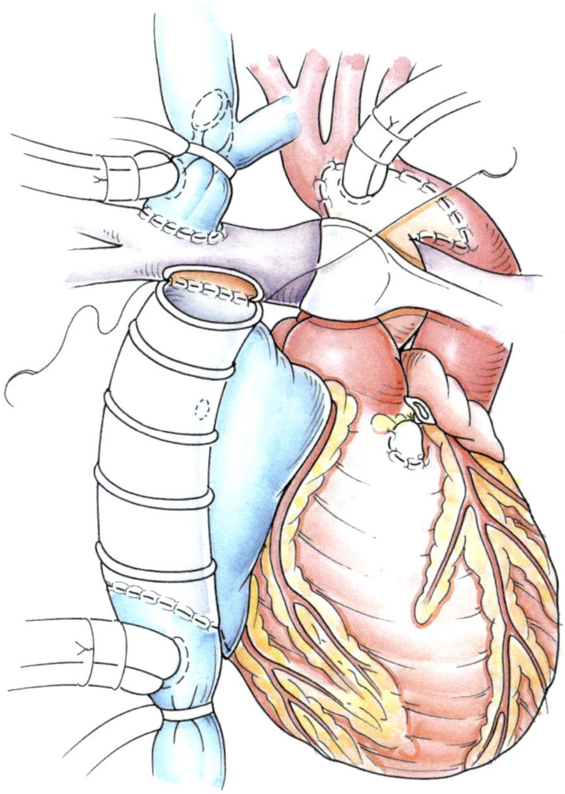

Fig. 28.2 Total cavopulmonary connection with extracardiac conduit: connecting extracardiac conduit with the inferior vena cava and right pulmonary artery respectively, suturing right atrial stump

of the atrial septal defect. It should be noted during suturing of the upper edge that the tunnel should connect both with the superior vena cava and with the pulmonary artery anastomosis (Fig. 28.5).

Having finished the intracardiac tunnel, the right atrial incision is closed with continuous sutures. Occupying nearly half of the atrium's tissues, the intracardiac tunnel might grow and expand alongside the baby's growth (Fig. 28.6).

After hemi-Fontan surgery is performed in the second stage Norwood surgery, a total cavopulmonary connection procedure with an intra-atrial lateral tunnel should always be performed in the third stage. A diversion port is left at the inner side of the lateral tunnel. Figure 28.7 shows the postoperative connection after the Stage III Norwood procedure. A new ascending aorta, which is connected with the right ventricle, is established by shaping the pulmonary artery and aorta with a supplement patch. The artificial vascular graft of the systemic to pulmonary artery Sano shunt has been divided in the Stage II Norwood operation. Oxygenated blood in left atrium flows into the single ventricular cavity through the enlarged atrial septum and the tricuspid valve. Superior and inferior vena caval blood flows into pulmonary circulation through the tunnels and the atrial-pulmonary anastomosis.

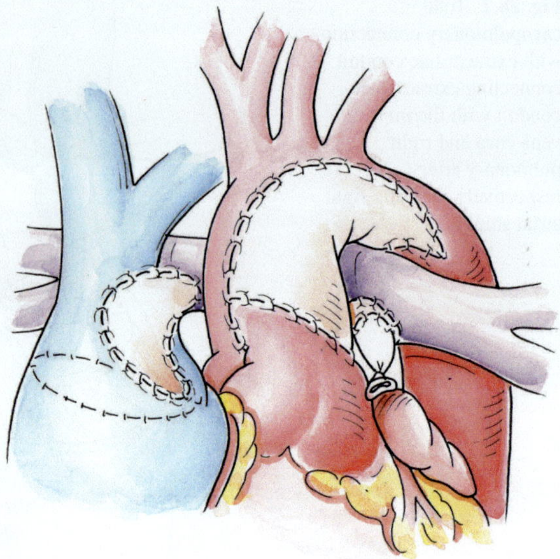

Fig. 28.3 Total cavopulmonary connection with intra-atrial lateral tunnel: schematic diagram after stage I Norwood surgery and hemi-Fontan surgery

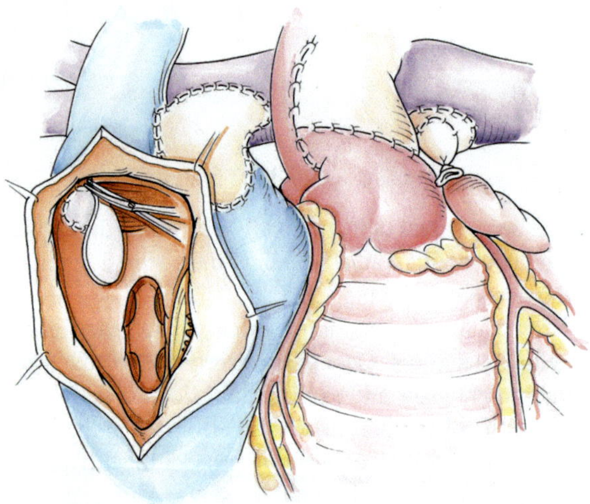

Fig. 28.4 Total cavopulmonary connection with intra-atrial lateral tunnel: cutting off Sano shunt vessel and pre-set patch

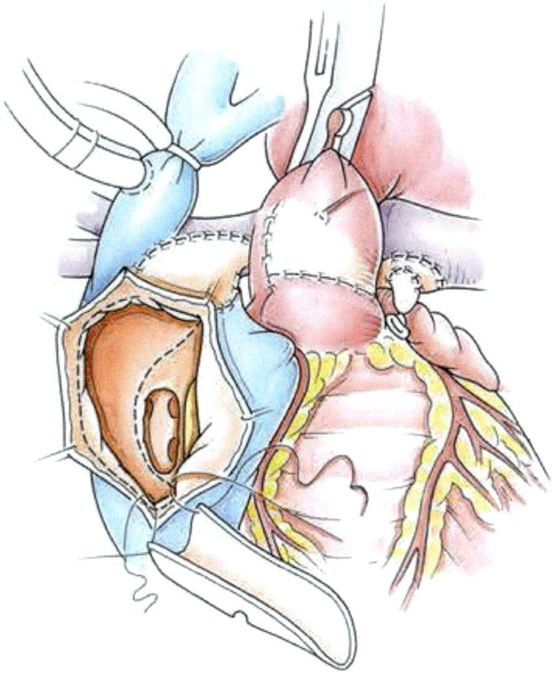

Fig. 28.5 Total cavopulmonary connection with intra-atrial lateral tunnel: implantation of tunnel patch with a hole in right atrium

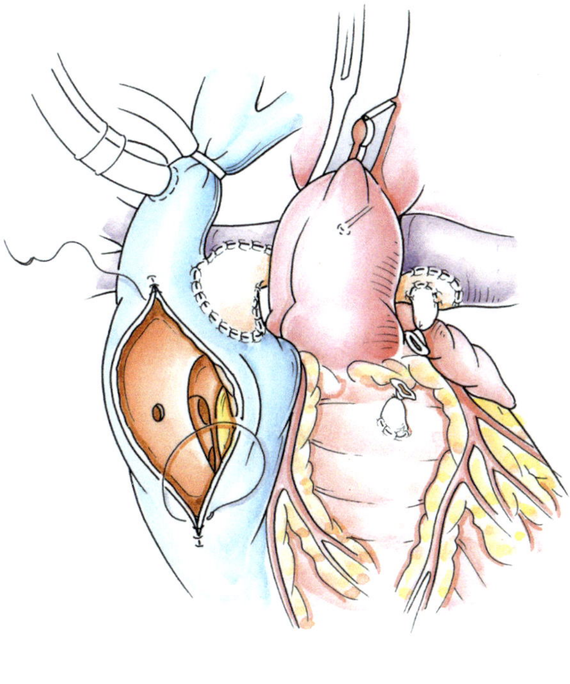

Fig. 28.6 Total cavopulmonary connection with intra-atrial lateral tunnel: suturing right atrium

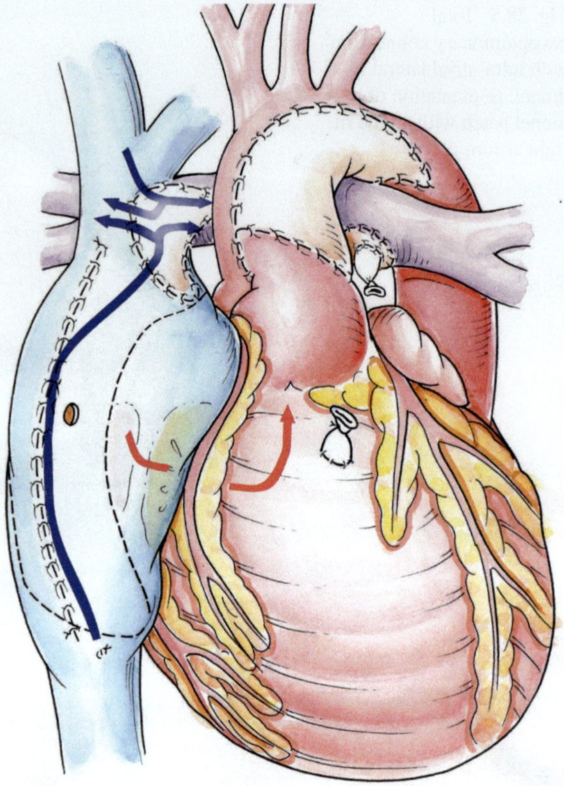

Fig. 28.7 Total cavopulmonary connection with intra-atrial lateral tunnel: the blood flow diagram after stage III Norwood surgery

Chapter 29
Stage I Norwood Procedure: Hybrid Therapy

Yu Guo Weng and Bin Qiao

Hybrid therapy can replace the Stage I Norwood procedure. It is especially suitable for patients with high-risk factors and for those who cannot undergo cardiopulmonary bypass, including cerebral hemorrhage, premature children, etc.

The hybrid treatment is performed in a hybrid operation room. The patient is supine with the median incision in the upper part of the sternum (Fig. 29.1).

The atrial septum is maximally dilated by a balloon catheter directed by transesophageal echocardiography through the foramen ovale or small atrial septal defect (Fig. 29.2).

The left and right pulmonary arteries are surrounded with polyester and tightened with forceps to 3 mm in diameter. Both the aortic pressure and blood oxygen saturation should be monitored. In the procedure, the pressure should be elevated, and the oxygen saturation should be maintained at the preoperative level, not less than 70%. Polyester ribbons are then fixed using Prolene sutures. If the oxygen saturation is too low, the bands across the left and right pulmonary arteries should be appropriately relaxed. The procedure should be performed after the hybridized treatment with the patient still on the operating table. Careful care should be taken to ensure that marginal arterial pressure and oxygen saturation are maintained for survival (Fig. 29.3).

Y. G. Weng (✉)
German Heart Center (Berlin), Berlin, Germany
e-mail: wengyuguo@dhzb.de

B. Qiao
Cardiovascular Institute, General Hospital of Jinan Military Region, Jinan, China

Cardiac Surgery Center, Western District of Shandong Provincial Hospital, Jinan, China

B. Qiao et al. (eds.), *Surgical Atlas of Functional Single Ventricle and Hypoplastic Left Heart Syndrome*, https://doi.org/10.1007/978-981-10-8435-5_29

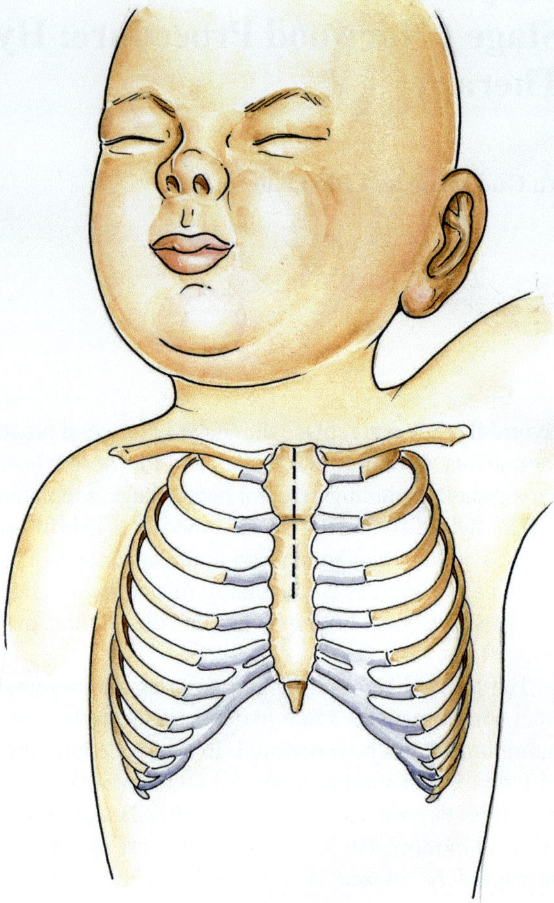

Fig. 29.1 Hybrid therapy of stage I Norwood procedure: splitting the upper part of the sternum

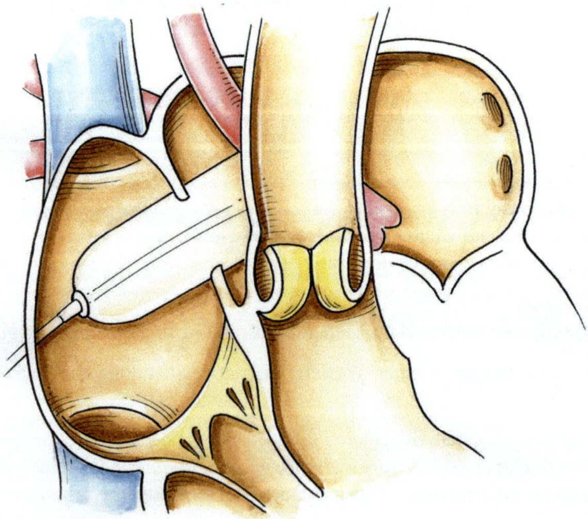

Fig. 29.2 Hybrid therapy of stage I Norwood procedure: enlargement of atrial septum with balloon catheter

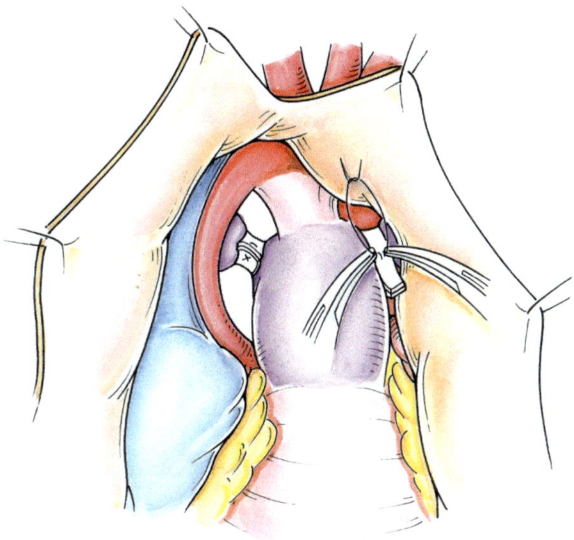

Fig. 29.3 Hybrid therapy of stage I Norwood procedure: banding the left and right pulmonary arteries

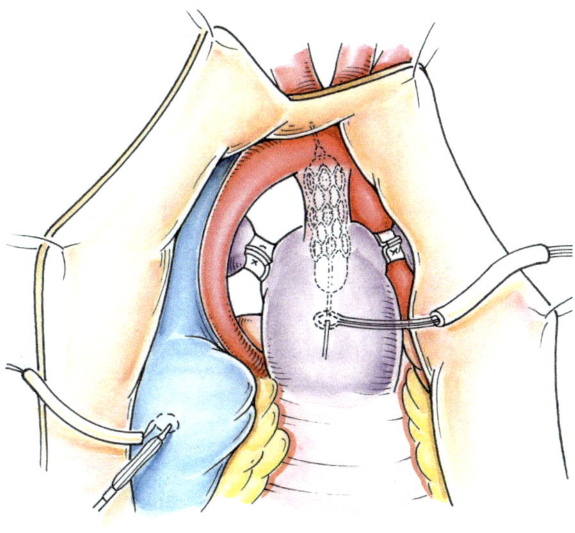

Fig. 29.4 Hybrid therapy of stage I Norwood procedure: intravascular stent implantation in PDA

An intravascular stent of suitable length and size is implanted in the patent ductus arteriosus through the purse string at the pulmonary trunk. This operation can also be performed before the constriction of the left and right pulmonary arteries has been fixed (Fig. 29.4).

This is a schematic diagram showing hybrid treatment instead of the first stage of Norwood surgery (Fig. 29.5).

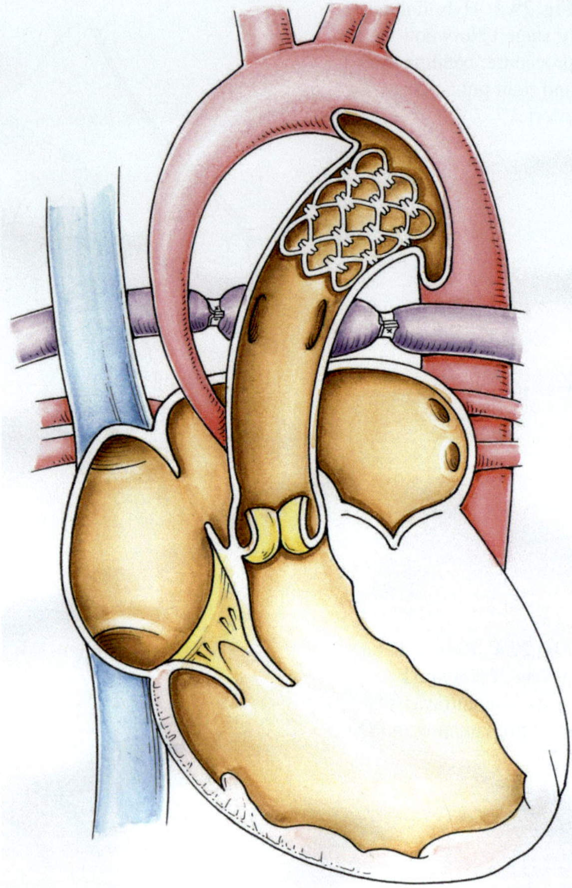

Fig. 29.5 Hybrid therapy of stage I Norwood procedure: schematic diagram after hybrid therapy

Chapter 30
Stage II Norwood Procedure After Hybrid Therapy: Hemi-Fontan and Bidirectional Glenn Shunt

Zhong Min Liu and Yu Guo Weng

The hybridization treatment of Stage I Norwood surgery simplifies surgical procedures, but succeeding work needs to be continually performed; for example, removal of the intravascular stent implanted in the ductus arteriosus, excision of ductus tissue and scar tissue resulting from stent implantation, handling possible stenosis of the pulmonary artery, and angioplasty and switch operations for the ascending aorta.

The operation should be carried out under cardiopulmonary bypass and subsequent deep hypothermic circulatory arrest. An aortic cannula is placed in the pulmonary artery main trunk, and a venous cannula is placed from the right atrium into the inferior vena cava using a bipolar single tube. The rubber bands preset across the left and right pulmonary arteries should be tightened immediately after the beginning of bypass to prevent lung perfusion. Cardiopulmonary bypass is stopped when rectal temperature reaches 18–20 °C. The innominate artery and the left carotid artery are then blocked, and cardiopulmonary bypass cannulas are removed. The dashed lines show the position of the main pulmonary artery transverse incision and filleting sites of the ascending aorta and aortic arch (Fig. 30.1).

Pulmonary artery main trunk and the hyperplastic arch are connected by the part of ascending aorta extracted from the allogeneic aortic graft. After division, the proximal and distal ends of the superior vena cava are anastomosed to the upper and lower surfaces of the right pulmonary artery, respectively. A transverse incision of the upper right atrium is made for suturing the patch, which separates blood flow from the inferior vena cava to the pulmonary artery. After the main trunk of the

Z. M. Liu (✉)
Shanghai Dongfang Hospital, Tongji University, Shanghai, China
e-mail: yuanzhang@easthospital.cn

Y. G. Weng
German Heart Center (Berlin), Berlin, Germany
e-mail: wengyuguo@dhzb.de

B. Qiao et al. (eds.), *Surgical Atlas of Functional Single Ventricle and Hypoplastic Left Heart Syndrome*, https://doi.org/10.1007/978-981-10-8435-5_30

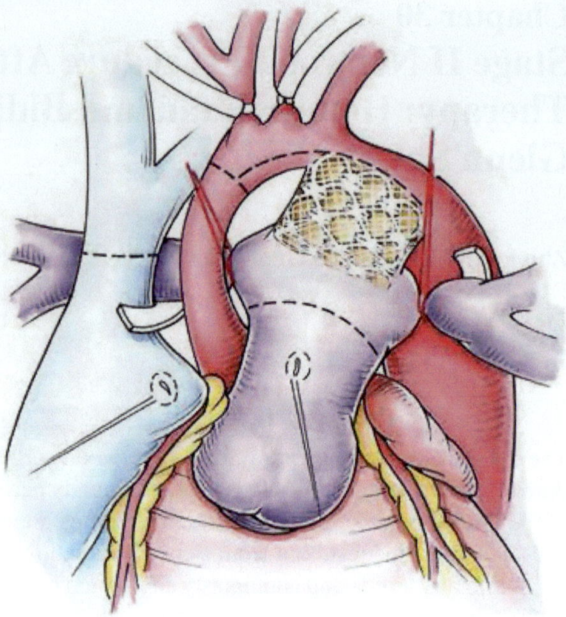

Fig. 30.1 Stage II Norwood procedure after hybrid therapy: the cutting site indicated as dashed line

pulmonary artery is transversely divided, the stent in the ductus arteriosus can be removed (Fig. 30.2).

The scar resulting from the tissue's reaction to stent implantation, and the ductus tissue itself, are all excised at the ductus end of pulmonary artery. The resulting incision is advised to be closed with a patch to ensure that there is no pulmonary artery stenosis (Fig. 30.3).

The distal end of the superior vena cava is anastomosed to the superior surface of the pulmonary artery, while its proximal end is anastomosed to the inferior surface (Fig. 30.4).

Meanwhile, the separating patch is placed in the right atrium through the divided superior vena cava or the right atrial venous intubation site. The pulmonary artery main trunk is anastomosed to the aortic allogeneic graft. The homograft is shaped to length and connected to the dysplastic arch. Finally, the small ascending aorta is end-to-side anastomosed to the neoaorta. Intubation, opening of bypass, and rewarming are successively performed. The hemi-Fontan operation is complete and ready for the Stage III Norwood procedure with cardiac lateral tunnel surgery, which can be accomplished by implanting the internal stent through the incised patch with an intervention method (Fig. 30.5).

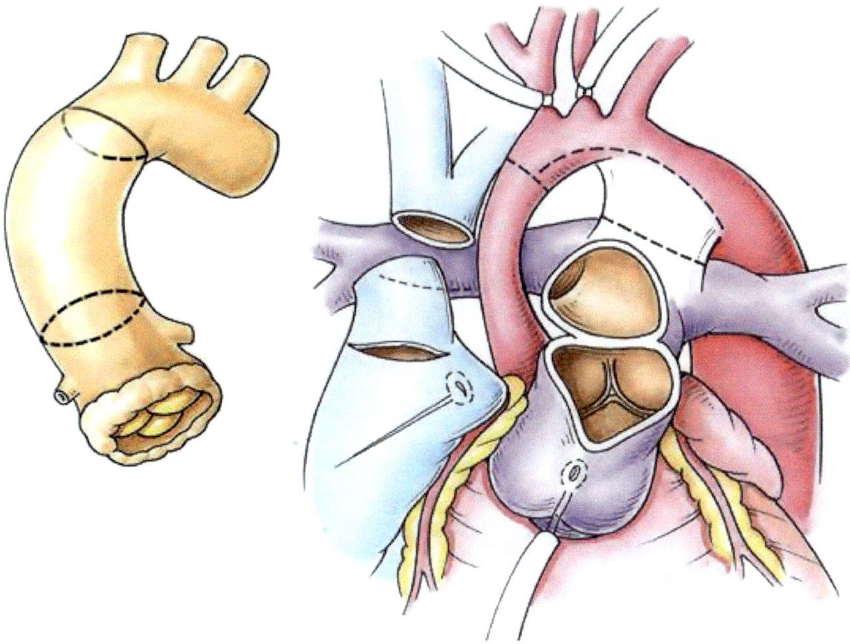

Fig. 30.2 Stage II Norwood procedure after hybrid therapy: fashioning the allogeneic aortic graft, transecting superior vena cava, making transverse incision at upper right atrium, transecting pulmonary artery trunk, and removing the ductus arteriosus stent

Fig. 30.3 Stage II Norwood procedure after hybrid therapy: closure of pulmonary artery at its ductus arteriosus end

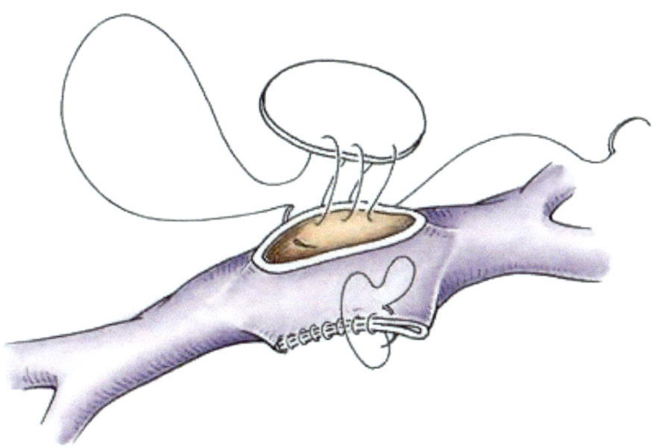

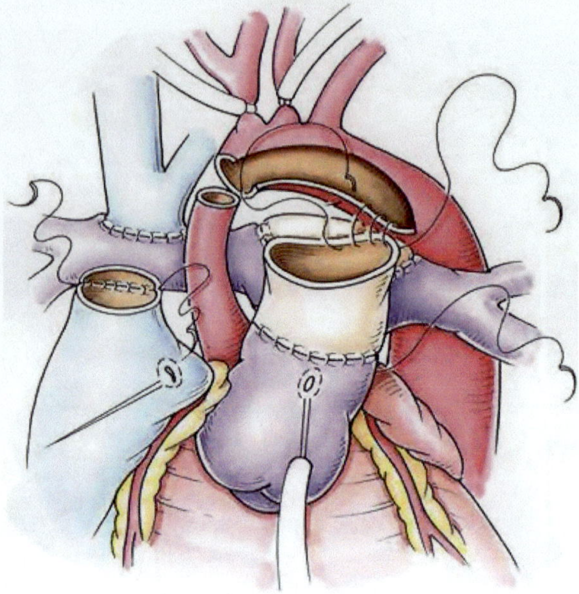

Fig. 30.4 Stage II Norwood procedure after hybrid therapy: anastomosing superior vena cava with right pulmonary artery at both its upper and lower wall

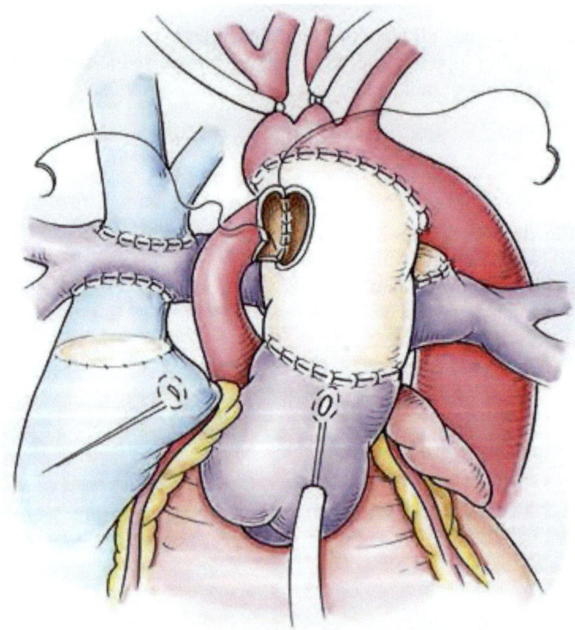

Fig. 30.5 Stage II Norwood procedure after hybrid therapy: suturing patch at the upper part of right atrium, anastomosing graft with fine ascending aorta

Bidirectional Glenn shunt surgery is relatively simple. Immediately after forming the new ascending aorta, circulation can be opened after re-intubation, followed by rewarming. The anastomosis of the superior vena cava to the right pulmonary artery is then performed. The time of deep hypothermic circulatory arrest can be cut in half (Fig. 30.6).

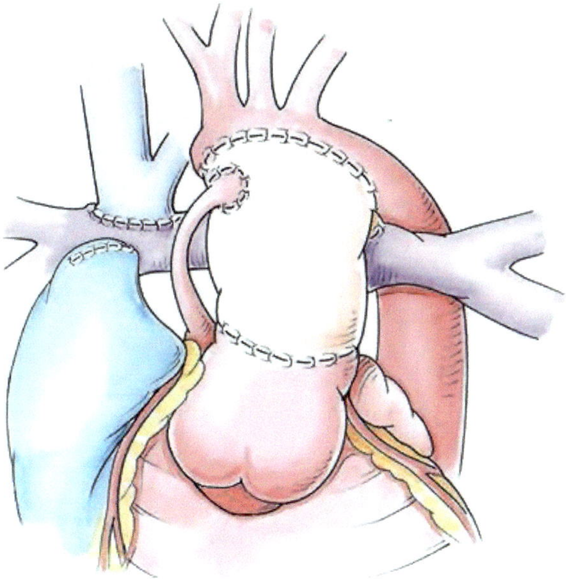

Fig. 30.6 Stage II Norwood procedure after hybrid therapy: bidirectional Glenn shunt performed after new aortic angioplasty

Chapter 31
Orthotopic Cardiac Transplantation for Left Ventricular Hypoplasia Syndrome

Zhong Min Liu and Yu Guo Weng

The hearts of patients with hyperplastic left heart syndrome are almost normal in size and smaller than the hearts of patients with dilated cardiomyopathy, so the heart of a brain-dead neonate with comparable size could be selected as a donor heart. A double atrium cardiac transplantation is the earliest classic technique. The operation method is relatively simple. However, there are four atria in total, two from the donor and the two of the recipient, in one patient after heart transplantation, so the post-operative atrium is accordingly enlarged. Because action between the inherent and the donor's sinoatrial nodes cannot maintain coordination, there is a possibility of electrophysiologic disturbances in the natural atrium. Arrhythmia is another potential complication because the right atrial anastomosis is much closer to the sinoatrial node, and because the donor's right atrium can be distorted due to a mismatch between the donor and recipient hearts. The bicaval heart transplantation, as its name suggests, is a technique to fashion a superior/inferior vena caval end-to-end anastomosis between the donor and recipient hearts during heart transplantation. In recent years, the bicaval technique has been widely adopted.

The cardiotomy should be performed under cardiopulmonary bypass and deep hypothermia. The pulmonary artery and inferior and superior venae cavae are cannulated. Tourniquets are placed across the innominate artery and left common carotid artery and tightened after arresting circulation and cutting the aortic arch to prevent air embolism. Rubber bands around the left and right pulmonary arteries are used to block the left and right pulmonary arteries when cardiopulmonary bypass has begun (Fig. 31.1).

Z. M. Liu (✉)
Shanghai Dongfang Hospital, Tongji University, Shanghai, China
e-mail: yuanzhang@easthospital.cn

Y. G. Weng
German Heart Center (Berlin), Berlin, Germany
e-mail: wengyuguo@dhzb.de

B. Qiao et al. (eds.), *Surgical Atlas of Functional Single Ventricle and Hypoplastic Left Heart Syndrome*, https://doi.org/10.1007/978-981-10-8435-5_31

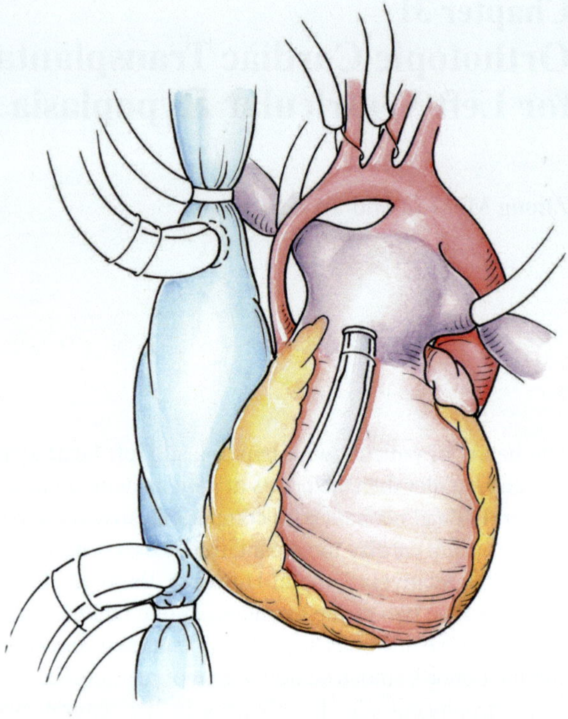

Fig. 31.1 Biatrial orthotopic heart transplantation: Establishment of cardiopulmonary bypass, blocking left and right pulmonary arteries

Under conditions of deep hypothermia circulatory arrest, the right atrium and then the left atrium is cut open along the interatrial sulci. After the pulmonary artery and the ascending aorta have been transected, the entire sick heart can be taken out. A porous left heart drainage tube (F12) should be placed into the right pulmonary vein to reduce the load of the donor heart. The edge of the right and left atrium is trimmed without preserving too many atrial tissues. The ascending aortic stump is sewn closed. The pulmonary arterial side of the ductus arteriosus is ligated, and side remains of ductus tissue are completely excised. The entire aortic arch is filleted to the normal size of the descending aorta (Fig. 31.2).

The ascending aorta, aortic arch, and proximal descending aorta should remain intact during recovery of the donor heart. After the donor heart arrives in the operating room, a part of the aortic arch and ascending aorta should be removed (Fig. 31.3).

The brachiocephalic, left common carotid artery, and left subclavian artery are excised from the donor heart (Fig. 31.4).

The fashioned donor heart arch (with part of the ascending aorta) is anastomosed to the hypoplastic arch with continuous sutures (Fig. 31.5).

Following completion of the anastomosis, the ascending aorta is cannulated with air-venting. The innominate artery and left common carotid artery are opened while the ascending aorta is blocked. Cardiopulmonary bypass is initiated, and rewarming is gradually performed (Fig. 31.6).

While warming, a series of procedures for the donor–recipient anastomosis can be performed. The procedures begin with the suturing of the posterior wall of the left

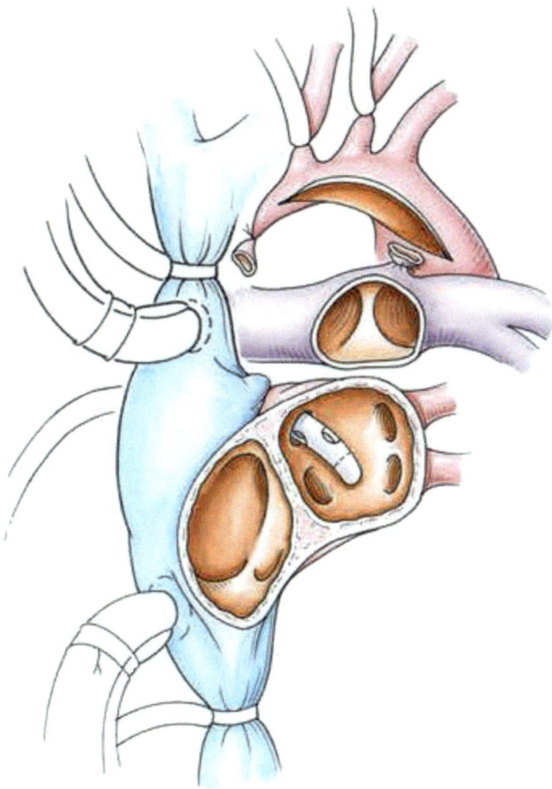

Fig. 31.2 Biatrial orthotopic heart transplantation: the heart removed, the stump of the ascending aorta sutured, the ductus arteriosus sutured, the small aortic arch cut

atrium, and the subsequent placement of a left heart drainage tube in the left ventricle through the mitral valve. Left atrium suturing is continued until completed. Left heart suction is stopped, followed by air-venting. Of note, before the ascending aorta of the donor heart is anastomosed, the left heart is in the opened state; if left heart suction ceases, the left atrium and left ventricle can be naturally filled with blood, and it is conducive to fully vent the left heart before opening circulation. When the donor heart is delivering and when the anastomosis is processing, the air has likely accumulated in all parts of the heart chamber, particularly in the right or left atrial appendage. The small air embolism would present in the coronary artery due to any tiny air bubbles and would consequently result in ischemia and dysfunction of the donor heart. The dashed line from the opening of the inferior vena cava toward the base of the right atrial appendage indicates that the right atrial incision lies far away from the sinoatrial node (Fig. 31.7).

The anastomosis of the left atrium ends in front of the atrial septum. The right atrium is cut open along the dotted line. As opposed to the left atrium, the right atrial anastomosis is initiated from the atrial septum. Starting from the inferior atrial septum, the posterior wall of the right atrium is upwardly anastomosed to the atrial septum of the left atrium and immediately followed by suturing of the anterior wall of the right atrium; the other end of suture line is continued forward from the right atrial inferior anastomosis, and knots should be tied at the anterior wall of the right atrium (Fig. 31.8).

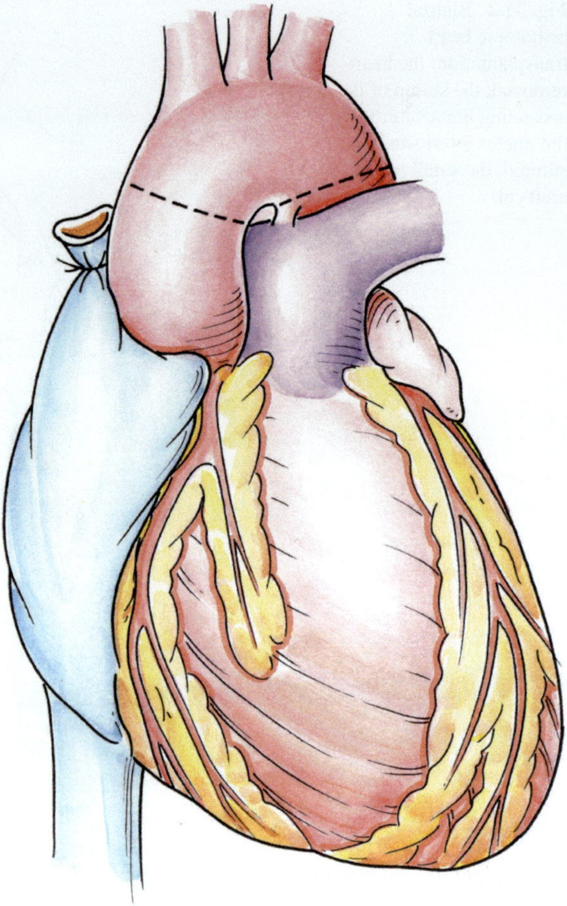

Fig. 31.3 Biatrial orthotopic heart transplantation: the part of the aortic arch and ascending aorta cut along dash line

The pulmonary artery anastomosis should be undertaken prior to tying knots in the right atrial anastomosis. It is relatively simple. The pulmonary artery anastomosis begins suturing from the posterior atrial wall and ties the suture at the anterior wall. 6-0 Prolene sutures are usually suitable for neonates (Fig. 31.9).

The ascending aorta is anastomosed last in the same fashion as the pulmonary artery. The sutures of choice depend on the size of the sick child. It is vital to vent air before tying knots. The venting is performed through an ordered series of actions: ceasing left heart suction, releasing inferior and superior vena caval tourniquets to fill the right heart with blood, relaxing of right atrial sutures not yet tied, and gently massaging and shaking the heart. Following right heart venting, the ascending aorta vent is started with a needle after the aortic sutures have been tied and the cross-clamp has been released. Meanwhile, the donor left heart is suctioned and drained, and the heart is continuously massaged. According to donor heart ischemia time guidelines, under effective low load conditions, left heart drainage can run in parallel for about 1 h. Left heart drainage is critical in pediatric and especially neonatal heart transplantation. Pediatric and neonatal hearts are sensitive to excessive left

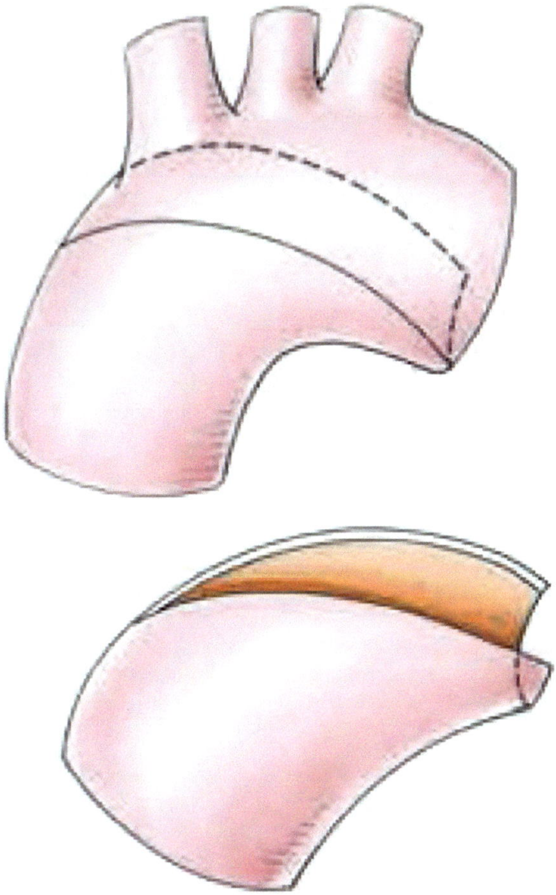

Fig. 31.4 Biatrial orthotopic heart transplantation: pruning the aortic arch of donor heart

ventricular volume overload due to lack of heart exercise. Excessive left heart expansion will impair its function, especially without a normal heartbeat. Therefore, left heart expansion should be avoided during the entire heart transplant process, as well as during donor heart recovery. Following left ventricular drainage, the CPB flow can be gradually reduced and cardiopulmonary bypass can be stopped while heart function is carefully inspected. Diluted adrenaline, instead of dopamine, to which pediatric cardiac contractive function is not very sensitive, can be dropped on the surface of the heart if necessary (Fig. 31.10).

The dashed line in Fig. 31.11 shows the line along which tissue is cut or removed from the sick heart. The CPB method is the same as in biatrial transplantation, except that the cannulas are placed at distal ends of the superior and inferior venae cavae. When the superior and inferior venae cavae are excised, a part of the right atrium remains, such that the caval anastomosis can be later expanded.

After resection of the sick heart, the remaining parts are shown in Fig. 31.12. A part of the atrial wall should be left in the superior/inferior vena cava. The left atrium above the mitral annulus should remain. The left atrial anastomosis should

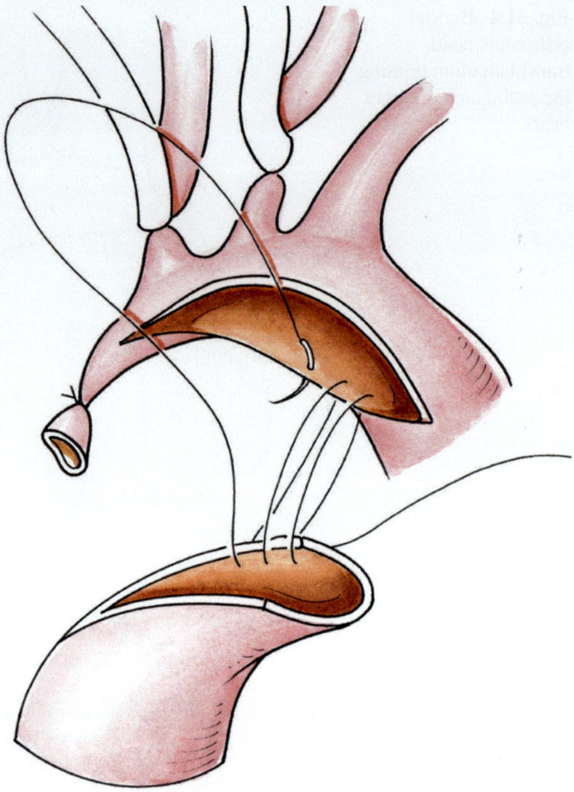

Fig. 31.5 Biatrial orthotopic heart transplantation: anastomosing the aorta arch of donor heart to the recipient one

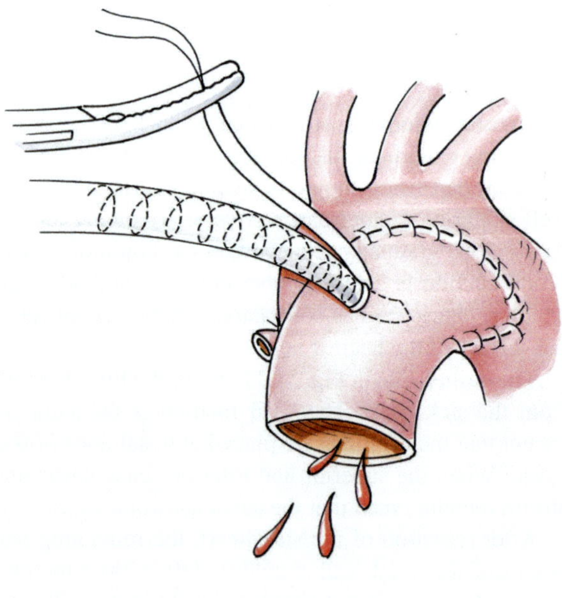

Fig. 31.6 Biatrial orthotopic heart transplantation: exhaust via ascending aorta, anonymous artery and left common carotid artery opened

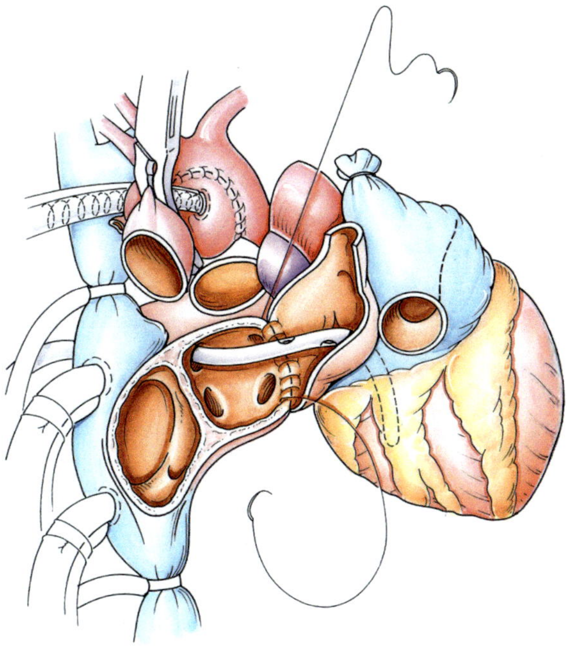

Fig. 31.7 Biatrial orthotopic heart transplantation: left atrial anastomosis

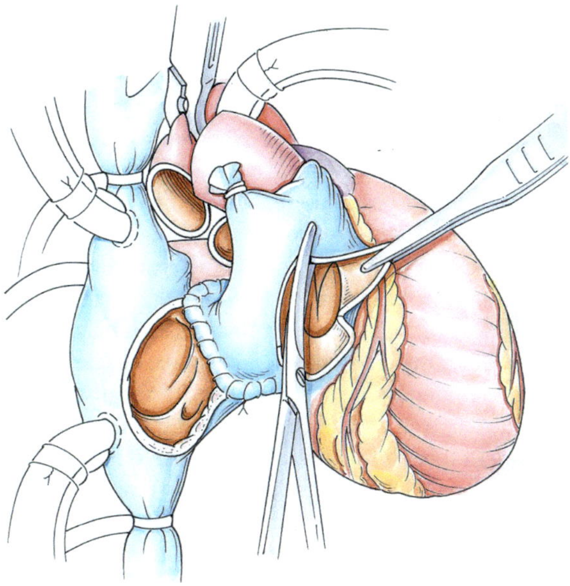

Fig. 31.8 Biatrial orthotopic heart transplantation: right atrial anastomosis

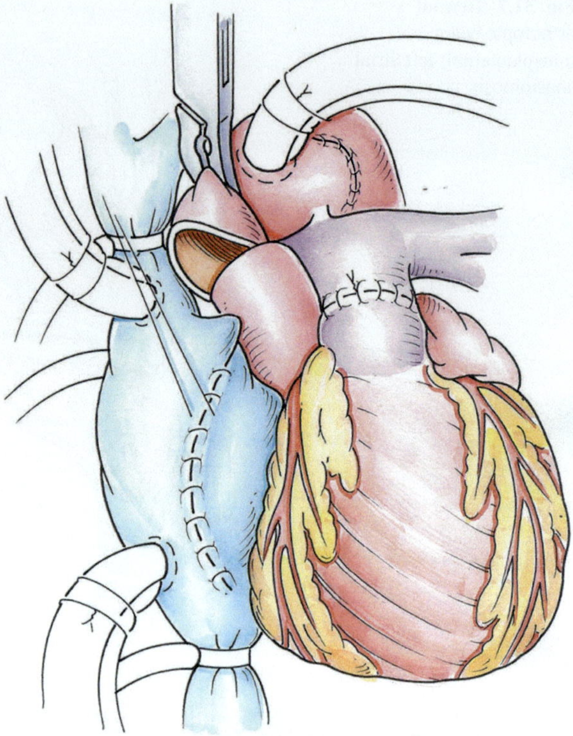

Fig. 31.9 Biatrial orthotopic heart transplantation: the main pulmonary artery anastomosis

be as large as possible. The normal pulmonary artery trunk should be kept large enough at its ductus end to facilitate suturing and division of the ductus. The small hypoplastic ascending aorta is oversewn at its distal end, and the rest can be excised along with the sick heart. The ductus tissue connected to the aorta should be removed, and the small aortic arch is filleted.

The aortic root is reconstructed using the donor heart aorta, as is the case in biatrial heart transplantation. Following reconstruction, a cannula is placed at the aorta. After the head vent, the ascending aorta is blocked, cardiopulmonary bypass is commenced, and slow rewarming is simultaneously started (Fig. 31.13).

The left atrial anastomosis is fashioned as described in Fig. 31.7, using continuous sutures starting from the left edge of the resulting atrial incision. The suturing is continued upward, and the two ends of the sutures are tied in the middle of the atrial septum. Before closing the left atrial anastomosis, the left heart drainage tube should be placed in the left ventricular cavity through the donor mitral valve. In bicaval heart transplantation, the entire length of the inferior and superior venae cavae should be intact when removing the donor heart. When trimming, surgeons should carefully check the integrity of the superior and inferior venae cavae and search for any damage. The caval incision should be smooth and tidy to facilitate anastomotic healing. An incision of 1–2 cm is made on each donor vena cava close to the interatrial sulci along the inferior and superior venae cavae to expand the connection of the recipient vena cava with a part of the atrial wall. Figure 31.14 shows that the

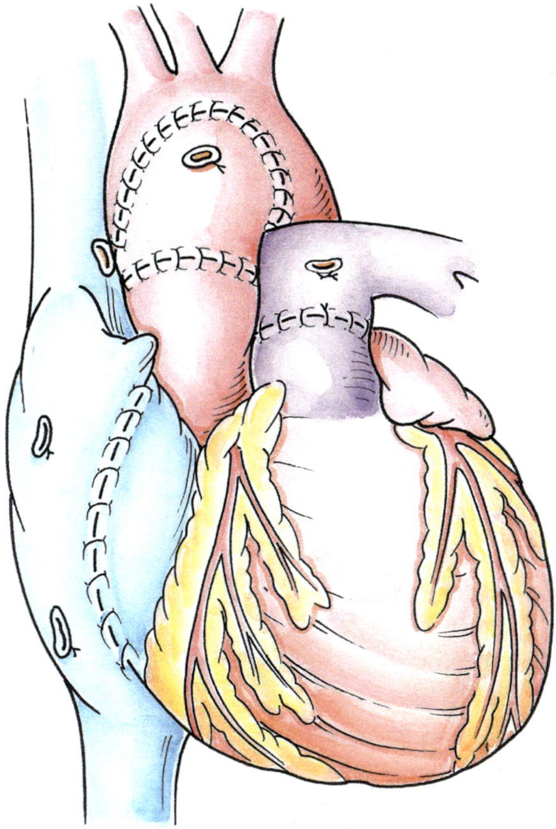

Fig. 31.10 Biatrial orthotopic heart transplantation: ascending aorta anastomosis, surgery completed

superior vena caval incision has been cut open; the dashed line is the incision line of the inferior vena cava.

After a successful heart transplantation, children grow quickly. Finer sutures are advised to be adopted to anastomose the donor heart to autologous tissue. They will be broken with growth of the anastomosis under chronic stress without adverse effects on the growth of the anastomosis. Potentially cicatricial stenosis may occur at the superior and inferior venae cavae due to resident low pressure. By using the inferior and superior venae cavae with residual atrial wall tissue from the recipient heart and with an expanded incision at the donor heart, the vena caval anastomosis can be sufficiently expanded with increasing capacity to avoid the presence of venous return resistance when patients grow. The superior vena caval anastomosis is performed first, followed by the inferior anastomosis. Figure 31.15 shows the anastomosing of the inferior vena cava with atrial wall to the incision at the inferior vena cava of the donor heart.

Finally, the anastomosis of the ascending aorta is performed. After completion of the heart transplantation, heart venting, cross-clamp opening, and left ventricular draining are routinely performed. With warming, parallel bypass is continued until the donor heart is able to independently sustain the circulatory system (Fig. 31.16).

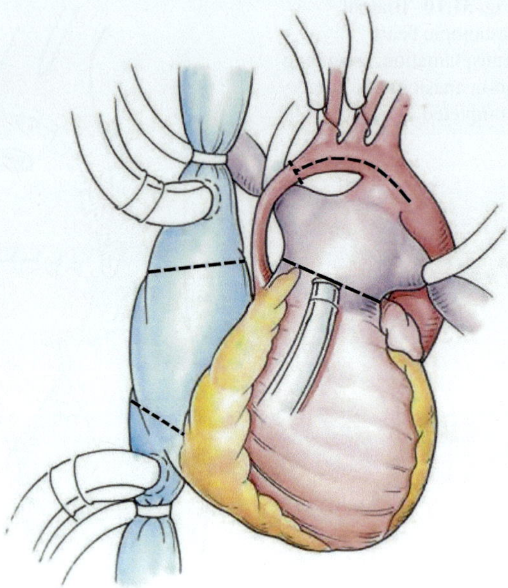

Fig. 31.11 Bicaval orthotopic heart transplantation: dashed line shows the cutting or removing position on sick heart

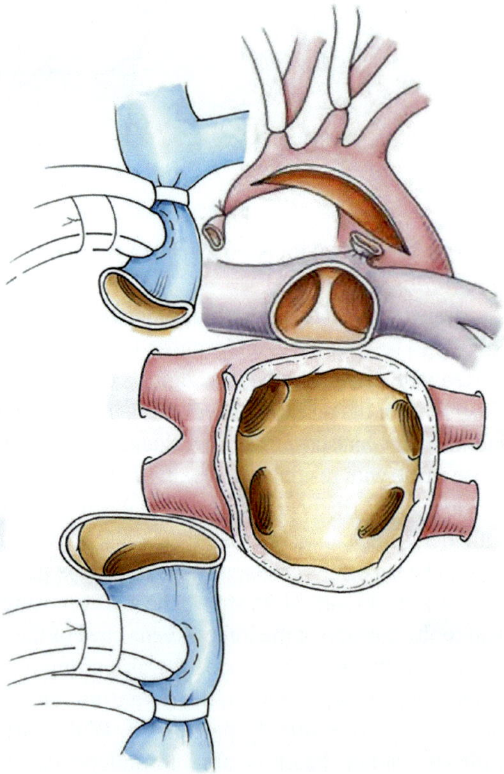

Fig. 31.12 Bicaval orthotopic heart transplantation: the remainder of the sick heart

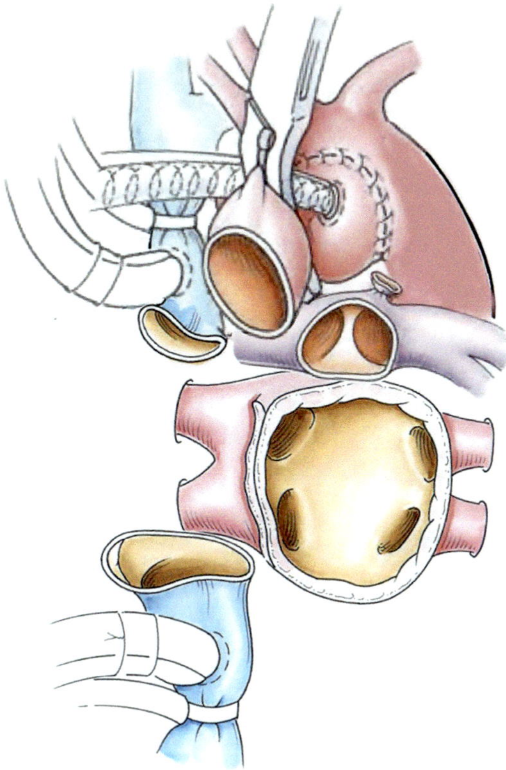

Fig. 31.13 Bicaval orthotopic heart transplantation: reconstruction of the aortic root

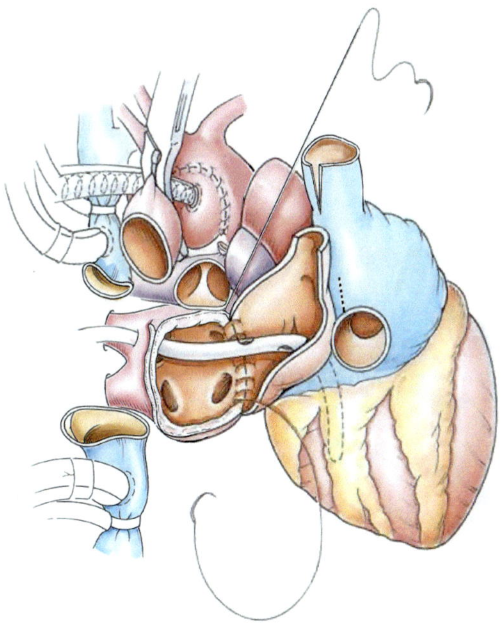

Fig. 31.14 Bicaval orthotopic heart transplantation: left atrial anastomosis

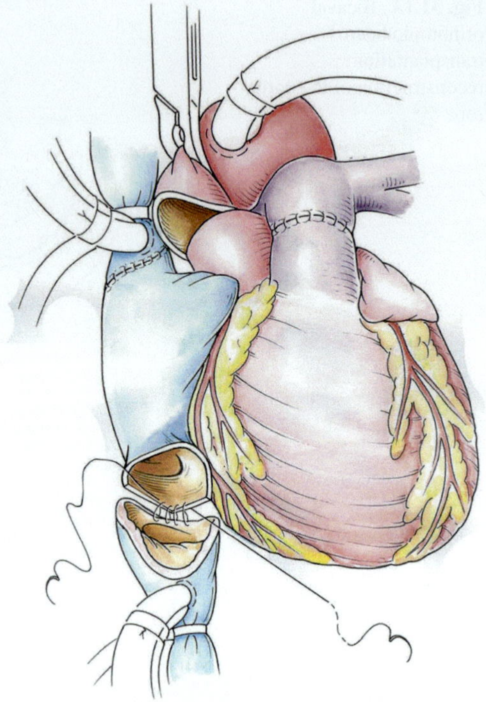

Fig. 31.15 Bicaval orthotopic heart transplantation: superior vena cava, inferior vena cava anastomosis

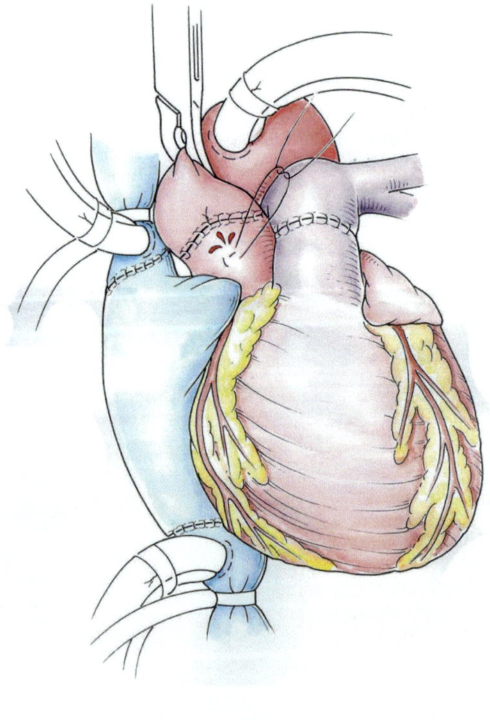

Fig. 31.16 Bicaval orthotopic heart transplantation: ascending aortic anastomosis

Chapter 32
Discussion

Yu Guo Weng, Bin Qiao, and Zhong Min Liu

32.1 Postoperative Treatment and Major Complications

The systemic and pulmonary circulations are still sustained by a single ventricle after the first stage Norwood procedure. Maintaining the required arterial pressure for systemic circulation and the oxygen saturation necessary for life are the keys to postoperative treatment. In early stages, if there is excessive pulmonary blood with oxygen saturation greater than 85% and a low arterial pressure is observed, it is necessary to increase pulmonary vascular resistance and pressure to reduce the pulmonary flow. A good example of increasing the resistance and pressure is to maintain 20% of oxygen inhalation and 30–40 mmHg of carbon dioxide partial pressure. A sufficient dose of milrinone can maintain venous pressure by dilating blood vessels, and a small amount of dopamine may have a dilating effect on the renal artery. Lower blood pressure can be treated with adrenaline doses ranging from 0.02 to 0.06 μg/kg/min. To treat metabolic acidosis, positive end expiratory pressure can be elevated with assisted ventilation. If excessive pulmonary blood is present due to an oversized systemic to pulmonary artery diversion, a constriction of the shunt blood vessels can be performed. If there is pulmonary blood with oxygen saturation less

Y. G. Weng (✉)
German Heart Center (Berlin), Berlin, Germany
e-mail: wengyuguo@dhzb.de

B. Qiao
Cardiovascular Institute, General Hospital of Jinan Military Region, Jinan, China

Cardiac Surgery Center, Western District of Shandong Provincial Hospital, Jinan, China

Z. M. Liu
Shanghai Dongfang Hospital, Tongji University, Shanghai, China
e-mail: yuanzhang@easthospital.cn

B. Qiao et al. (eds.), *Surgical Atlas of Functional Single Ventricle and Hypoplastic Left Heart Syndrome*, https://doi.org/10.1007/978-981-10-8435-5_32

than 70%, pure oxygen overventilation can be given to drive carbon dioxide partial pressure below 30 mmHg; the pulmonary vessel is dilated to decrease its resistance. Adrenaline drugs can also be applied to increase systemic resistance, thereby increasing the blood flow to the lungs. However, if the bodily circulation resistance is less than 65 mmHg and carbon dioxide partial pressure is less than 20 mmHg, the bodily pulmonary artery anastomosis is likely small, and the prognosis of conservative treatment is poor. A dose of 10 mg/kg of aspirin has been given at many centers to avoid an embolism in the shunt. Of note, however, nearly 26% of patients with congenital heart disease have aspirin resistance. After the first stage of the Norwood procedure, the ideal oxygen saturation is approximately 75%, indicating that the blood flow ratio of pulmonary to systemic circulation is less than one. Other common complications, including arrhythmia and low cardiac output, may be related to insufficient retrograde perfusion of the coronary artery through the formed ascending aorta and aortic arch.

Arterial pressure, venous pressure, and oxygen saturation should be monitored after Fontan surgery. The primary measures of postoperative treatment are the reduction of pulmonary vascular resistance, the maintenance of proper respiratory alkalosis, and early warfarin anticoagulation. Adrenaline should be given at 0.02–0.06 g/kg/min to deal with early postoperative low cardiac output. Dopamine has little effect on neonatal myocardial contractility but plays a role in renal artery dilatation. Milrinone can be used to maintain venous pressure. However, large doses of myocardial contractile agents also increase the resistance of the pulmonary arteries, so the reduction of pulmonary arterial resistance is preferable in elevating oxygen saturation. Arrhythmia and bradycardia can affect pulmonary blood flow, so a pacemaker should be placed if needed. Arrhythmia is a common complication after a Fontan operation, which is a likely result of damage to the sinoatrial node during surgery and especially atrial enlargement after surgery. To treat metabolic acidosis, positive end expiratory pressure should be elevated by using a ventilator. Late complications include hypoproteinemia, ascites, pleural effusion, and systemic edema. Stenosis of the passage from the systemic vein to the pulmonary artery, as well as blood vortex and blood stagnation in the pipeline, can also contribute to eventual Fontan surgery failure. If the child does not have any heart transplant contraindications, the only subsequent consideration is heart transplantation.

The primary treatment after heart transplantation is anti-immune therapy; the triple immunosuppressive agents of cyclosporine, glucocorticoid, and azathioprine or MMF should be routinely applied for antirejection reactions. Anti-immune induction can be performed by intravenously infusing methylprednisolone at 10 mg/kg at the beginning of cardiopulmonary bypass. After heart transplantation, rejection reactions are always the main threat; life-long anti-immune therapy is required. Pediatric hypertension is a more common complication, as is the case with heart transplantation for other diseases. Renal impairment, lymphomas or other tumors, and coronary artery and other vascular lesions can present as survival time increases.

32.2 Efficacy

32.2.1 Stage I Norwood Procedure Effect

32.2.1.1 Survival Rate

The surgical results of 198 neonates reported by Children's Hospital of Philadelphia show a hospital mortality rate of about 28% and an 18-month survival rate of 61% after the first stage Norwood procedure. According to an analysis of 294 cases that underwent the Norwood surgery in a number of US hospitals in 1985, the overall early mortality rate was 70% (174/249), the disability rate was 91% (101/111) in hospitals that has less than 16 surgical cases, and the mortality rate was 53% (73/138) in hospitals that conducted more than 35 surgical cases annually. Studies have shown that the surgical survival rate of HLHS after the first stage Norwood has continued to rise in recent years, and effective postoperative care is critically important for improving the survival rate (Tweddell et al. 2002). The survival rate reached 85% out of 100 cases with HLHS that underwent the first stage Norwood operation at the University of Michigan between 2000 and 2002. According to the database of the American Association of Thoracic Surgery Physicians, the survival rate of 2320 patients with HLHS after the first stage palliative procedure was 81.4%.

32.2.1.2 Risk Factors for Surgery

(1) Above 1 month of age, severe pulmonary hypertension, premature infants below 35 weeks of gestation, weight below 2.5 kg, operation time too early (less than 4 days) or too late (more than 14 days), and other combined abnormalities; (2) preoperative situation: severe brucellosis patients with a serious imbalance in the ratio of body to lung circulation, insufficient systemic perfusion, refractory metabolic acidosis, hypotension, and obstruction of venous flow return; (3) anatomical factors: aortic and mitral valve atresia with ascending aorta diameter less than 2–3 mm.

Too small an ascending aorta (less than 2 mm in diameter) may be an important risk factor for late postoperative death. Moderate to severe tricuspid insufficiency is associated with postoperative death, while a low pH value of preoperative arterial blood is not a risk factor for postoperative death because it can be preoperatively corrected to normal levels.

32.2.1.3 Hemodynamics and Morphological Results

Computer-aided hydrodynamic techniques can be employed to study postoperative hemodynamics. There were only 400 cases with a pressure gradient above 4 mmHg when unlimited atrial traffic was constructed by atrial septum dissection. Approximately 10% of cases had developed late postoperative tricuspid insufficiency in grades III to IV. There was little pressure gradient between the right ventricle and the reconstructed ascending aorta. The size of the aortic arch was normally manifested by angiography, but there were still 10–15% of cases with distal aortic arch stenosis and a systolic pressure gradient greater than 25 mmHg. In a 1-year follow-up after surgery, Qp/Qs was 0.8–1.5 in most cases, and the pulmonary vascular resistance index was above 4 Wood units/m^2 in 15–20% of patients. Pulmonary artery distortions occurred in 12% of patients, and right ventricular end diastolic pressure was above 12 mmHg in 10% of patients.

32.2.2 Stage I Hybrid Surgery Effect

32.2.2.1 Survival Rate

The time-dependent survival rate of hybridization therapy included the survival rate between staged operations, and the survival rate after the completed correction, which was 60%. Aortic arch retrograde obstruction due to the implantation of a ductus stent for aortic atresia patients may affect the survival rate. Akintuerk et al. reported that the survival rate was 83% when patients with HLHS underwent hybrid therapy instead of the first stage of Norwood surgery, and the mortality rate was 21% after two-stage corrective procedures (Akintuerk et al. 2002; Akintürk et al. 2007). The results were consistent with the reports of Galantowicz (Galantowicz and Cheatham 2005; Galantowicz et al. 2008). Although the number of cases of hybridization research has been relatively small, it has been reported that the incidence of complications after hybridization in children with HLHS is relatively high and may be associated with insufficient perfusion of the brain and coronary arteries caused by stenosis of the aorta.

32.2.2.2 Postoperative Risk Factor

Aortic atresia combined with aortic arch compulsory reflux may be an important risk factor for hybrid therapy.

32.2.3 Stage II Norwood Surgical Effect

Multicenter data analyzed by Jacobs showed that the mortality rate of the bidirectional cavopulmonary connection was approximately 5%. Since the physical status of children after the second stage correction has been significantly improved, the mortality rate during perioperative care and before Fontan surgery is usually very low.

32.2.4 *Fontan Surgical Effect*

32.2.4.1 Survival Rate

According to the Children's Hospital of Philadelphia's report on 50 patients that underwent a staged Fontan operation, the mortality rate was 16%. Jacobs reported that a total of 223 cases that underwent the single Fontan between 1985 and 1989 had a mortality rate of 16% (36 cases); a total of 200 cases (63% with HLHS, 127 cases) that underwent staged Fontan surgery between 1990 and 1993 had a mortality rate of 8%. The mortality rate of 112 cases was 4.5%; 36 of these cases had a fenestration, while 76 had a partial hepatic vein shunt. It is now generally agreed upon that staged Fontan surgery is safer than a single Fontan operation. The postoperative 4-year survival rate of modified Fontan surgery was 52%. Data from 2002 to 2006 has shown that the 5-year survival rate of neonates with HLHS after a staged correction can reach 50–70%.

32.2.4.2 Risk Factors of Surgery

Risk factors of the modified Fontan procedure include early performance (less than 3 months) of the Stage II Norwood procedure, postoperative arrhythmia, severe tricuspid insufficiency, which is likely to increase postoperative mortality, and a sudden reduction in ventricular capacity after the Fontan procedure.

32.2.4.3 Factors for Improved Surgical Outcome

(1) The overall operative technique has been improved; (2) A small diameter artificial homograft is selected for the shunt. A 4 mm diameter homograft for patients weighing more than 3.5 kg, 3–3.5 mm for those less than 3.5 kg, and a Blalock–Taussig shunt for those less than 2.5 kg; (3) To avoid left pulmonary artery compression and distortion, the aortic patch is chosen to be as small as possible. At present, some people perform the modified Norwood procedure without a patch; (4) To ensure good coronary perfusion, the angulated distortion of the aorta, pulmonary artery, and their anastomosis is avoided; (5) Fontan surgery is completed in two stages.

32.2.5 *Heart Transplantation Effect*

Rome Linda University Medical Center in the United States first reported out of 14 young cases, 11 survived cardiac transplantation. Long-term follow-up time was 3 years, while the maximum follow-up time was 5 years. Antirejection therapy for these patients was not any more complicated than for adults; the patients were treated with cyclosporine, azathioprine, etc. A total of 636 cases with HLHS were enrolled in affiliated hospitals of 40 universities in the United States from 1989 to 1993. Of these patients, 374 (59%) were not treated with any surgery, and 222 (35%) were treated with Norwood surgery, with a hospital mortality rate of 53%; a total of 40 cases (6.3%) were treated with heart transplantation with a hospital mortality rate of 42%. Bailey has received 176 patients with HLHS for 10 years since the first allogeneic heart transplantation was performed (Bailey 1985). Of these, 34 cases died while waiting for surgery (19%), and 142 cases had a heart transplant performed, with an operative mortality rate of 9% and long-term mortality rate of 15%. The operative survival rates at 1, 5, and 7 years were 84%, 76%, and 70%, respectively. Immune rejection caused more than half of the long-term deaths. Chrisant et al. reported that the 3-month mortality rate of multicenter HLHS children was 68%, and that the 5-year mortality rate was 54%, while waiting for and undergoing heart transplantation (Chrisant et al. 2005).

Heart transplantation is a one-time anatomical corrective procedure with a simple surgical technique and a favorable treatment outcome. However, because it is limited by the acquisition of donor hearts and other issues, such as long-term immune rejection and medication, it is not easy to popularize. Almond et al. reported that infants and young children waiting for a heart transplant in the United States have had a high mortality rate (17%) in the past two decades (Almond et al. 2009).

32.3 Conclusion and Evaluation

HLHS patients can only survive for a few days or weeks, therefore, must be treated immediately after birth, even though there is no radical surgery available. Heart transplantation is undoubtedly the most effective and reliable surgery; however, a newborn allogenic donor heart is almost impossible to obtain. For children who are so fortunate to get a donor heart, life-long anti-immune therapy is required after transplantation. Currently, the three-stage corrective surgery is an effective method. The ultimate therapeutic goal is to perform a total cavopulmonary connection (Fontan surgery) based on methods of treating functional single ventricle. If the treatment is successfully performed, right ventricular function should be shifted into left ventricular function, the pulmonary artery should be transposed into the aorta, and a systemic to pulmonary artery shunt should be established. Although the Fontan procedure has been widely carried out in addressing functional single ventricle with operative survival rates increasing, various postoperative complications often occur in the 10 years after the surgery, such as cavopulmonary anastomotic stenosis, thrombosis formation, arrhythmia, protein loss, and circulatory and systemic failure (failing Fontan). A range of factors for a successful treatment should be considered, such as the preparation for surgery after birth, three operations between 1 and 2 years of age, perioperative circulation management and systemic function support, feeding difficulties, and great psychological pressure.

The number of cases that have successfully undergone the Norwood staged procedure is increasing. About 70% of children with HLHS can live to adulthood after the corrective surgery. However, there are still many considerations of various aspects to take into account in addition to the complications of Fontan surgery, including intelligence, nerves, physical fitness, etc. These problems may result from multiple extracorporeal circulation surgeries, deep hypothermic circulatory arrest, as well as from hereditary factors and combinations of other congenital malformations. A successful palliative surgery depends on the technical strength of a hospital, which needs to have a neonatal or pediatric cardiology department, as well as senior pediatric cardiac surgeons. Other risk factors associated with pediatric treatment include low birth weight, other genetic syndromes, small atrial septal defects, and sudden closure of the patent ductus arteriosus. Excluding these risk factors, the 5-year survival rate may be close to 80%, but early surgical survivors represent varying degrees of developmental delay disability, which are aggravated as the patient ages. Follow-up data from the Berlin Heart Center shows that the incidence of postoperative developmental and behavioral disorders is higher in children than in the general population.

In our current clinical experience, surgical treatment of HLHS is unsatisfactory, regarding both the surgical mortality and long-term survival rates. Several operations are involved in the entire treatment process, which are expensive and time-consuming. Additionally, patients suffer from postoperative physical, mental, and personality disorders. In this case, some doctors have proposed the concept of "humanistic care" rather than surgery, which would lead to the death of neonates usually 2 weeks after birth. It cannot be carried out until the supervision of ethical and specialized personnel, such as physicians, psychologists, and lawyers, has been established to help the patient's relatives in making a decision.

References

Akintuerk H, Michel-Behnke I, Valeske K, Mueller M, Thul J, Bauer J, Hagel K-J, Kreuder J, Vogt P, Schranz D. Stenting of the arterial duct and banding of the pulmonary arteries. Basis for combined Norwood stage I and II repair in hypoplastic left heart. Circulation. 2002;105(9):1099–103. https://doi.org/10.1161/hc0902.104709.

Akintürk H, Michel-Behnke I, Valeske K, Mueller M, Thul J, Bauer J, Hagel K-J, Schranz D. Hybrid transcatheter–surgical palliation. Pediatr Cardiol. 2007;28(2):79–87. https://doi.org/10.1007/s00246-006-1444-7.

Almond CSD, Thiagarajan RR, Piercey GE, Gauvreau K, Blume ED, Bastardi HJ, Fynn-Thompson F, Singh TP. Waiting list mortality among children listed for heart transplantation in the United States. Circulation. 2009;119(5):717–27. https://doi.org/10.1161/CIRCULATIONAHA.108.815712.

Bailey LL. Role of cardiac replacement in the neonate. J Heart Transplant. 1985;4(5):506–9.

Chrisant MRK, Naftel DC, Drummond-Webb J, Chinnock R, Canter CE, Boucek MM, Boucek RJ, Hallowell SC, Kirklin JK, Morrow WR. Fate of infants with hypoplastic left heart syndrome listed for cardiac transplantation: a multicenter study. J Heart Lung Transplant. 2005;24(5):576–82. https://doi.org/10.1016/j.healun.2004.01.019.

Galantowicz M, Cheatham JP. Lessons learned from the development of a new hybrid strategy for the management of hypoplastic left heart syndrome. Pediatr Cardiol. 2005;26(2):190–9. https://doi.org/10.1007/s00246-004-0962-4.

Galantowicz M, Cheatham JP, Phillips A, Cua CL, Hoffman TM, Hill SL, Rodeman R. Hybrid approach for hypoplastic left heart syndrome: intermediate results after the learning curve. Ann Thorac Surg. 2008;85(6):2063–71. https://doi.org/10.1016/j.athoracsur.2008.02.009.

Tweddell JS, Hoffman GM, Mussatto KA, Fedderly RT, Berger S, Jaquiss RDB, Ghanayem NS, Frisbee SJ, Litwin SB. Improved survival of patients undergoing palliation of hypoplastic left heart syndrome: lessons learned from 115 consecutive patients. Circulation. 2002;106(12 suppl 1):I-82–9. https://doi.org/10.1161/01.cir.0000032878.55215.bd.

Part III
Image-Based Computational Simulation for Single Ventricle Hemodynamics and Its Clinical Applications

Image-based computational simulation (ICS) is progressively making its way from engineering and industrial applications to the clinical field as a promising tool to understand hemodynamics in the cardiovascular system. Advancements in ICS can be attributed to rapid development of medical imaging technology, computer techniques, and numerical methods of fluid dynamics. Since Dubini et al. (1996) first used ICS to investigate the hemodynamics of an idealized TCPC model, it has been utilized in many studies related to single ventricle surgeries, which involve TCPC, bidirectional Glenn, systemic-pulmonary shunt, tetralogy of Fallot, etc. ICS has the following three advantages:

It is a patient-specific noninvasive approach that greatly augments knowledge gained from in vivo or/and in vitro measurements.

It provides three-dimensional data that is not easily accessible for measurement or visualization.

It evaluates hemodynamic, biomechanical, and mechanobiological quantities which are otherwise difficult, if not impossible, to measure in vivo or/and in vitro.

This part will demonstrate the standard procedure of ICS for single ventricle patients and its clinical applications.

Reference

Dubini G, de Leval MR, Pietrabissa R, Montevecchi FM, Fumero R. A numerical fluid mechanical study of repaired congenital heart defects. Application to the total cavopulmonary connection. J Biomech. 1996;29(1):111–21. https://doi.org/10.1016/0021-9290(95)00021-6.

Chapter 33
Fundamentals of Image-Based Computational Simulation

Ajit P. Yoganathan and Zhenglun Alan Wei

The ICS technique revolves around principles of computational fluid dynamics (CFD) and medical imaging.

33.1 Image Acquisition and Processing

The standard procedure shown in Fig. 33.1 consists of three major steps: Image Acquisition, Image Processing, and Numerical Simulation. The purpose of image acquisition is primarily to acquire medical images for the reconstruction of patient-specific anatomy and flow data in blood vessels. The minimum requirement for a good anatomical reconstruction is a stack of high-resolution computer tomography (CT) or magnetic resonance (MR) images. Four images of a stack of axial CT acquisition are shown in Fig. 33.2.

Physiological flow data often includes flow rate, pressure, and systemic and/or pulmonary resistance, which are obtained from through-plane phase contrast MR (pcMR) imaging, dual-source CT, cardiac catheterization, and echocardiography (Fig. 33.3).

Acquired images are usually stored using the Digital Imaging and Communications in Medicine (DICOM) file format for communication between clinicians and engineers. Many commercial medical image processing software and image processing algorithms can be used to reconstruct in vivo patient-specific 3D anatomies (as shown in Fig. 33.4) and flow quantities (Frakes et al.

A. P. Yoganathan (✉) · Z. A. Wei
Wallace H. Coulter Department of Biomedical Engineering, Georgia Institute of Technology and Emory University, Atlanta, GA, USA
e-mail: ajit.yoganathan@bme.gatech.edu

B. Qiao et al. (eds.), *Surgical Atlas of Functional Single Ventricle and Hypoplastic Left Heart Syndrome*, https://doi.org/10.1007/978-981-10-8435-5_33

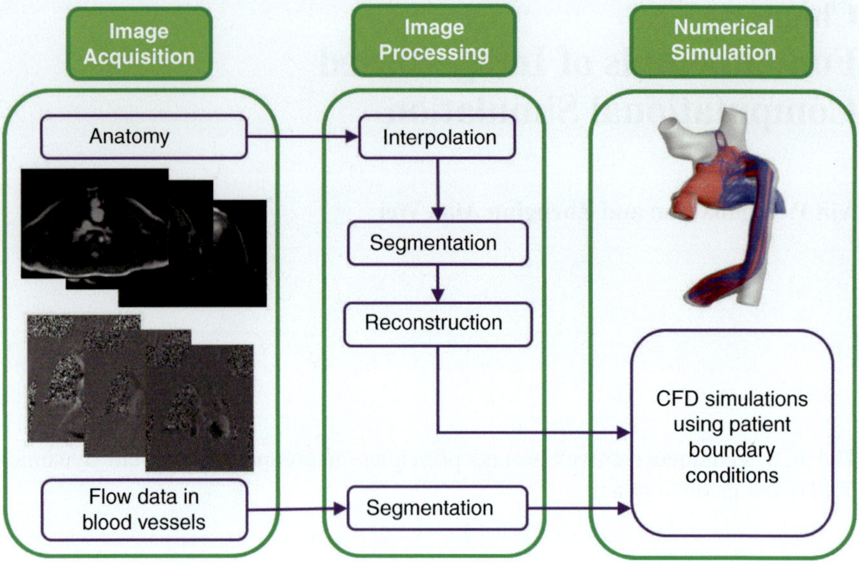

Fig. 33.1 A schematic drawing of the standard procedure for conducting image-based computational simulation for single ventricle patients [reproduced from Wei et al. (2017)]

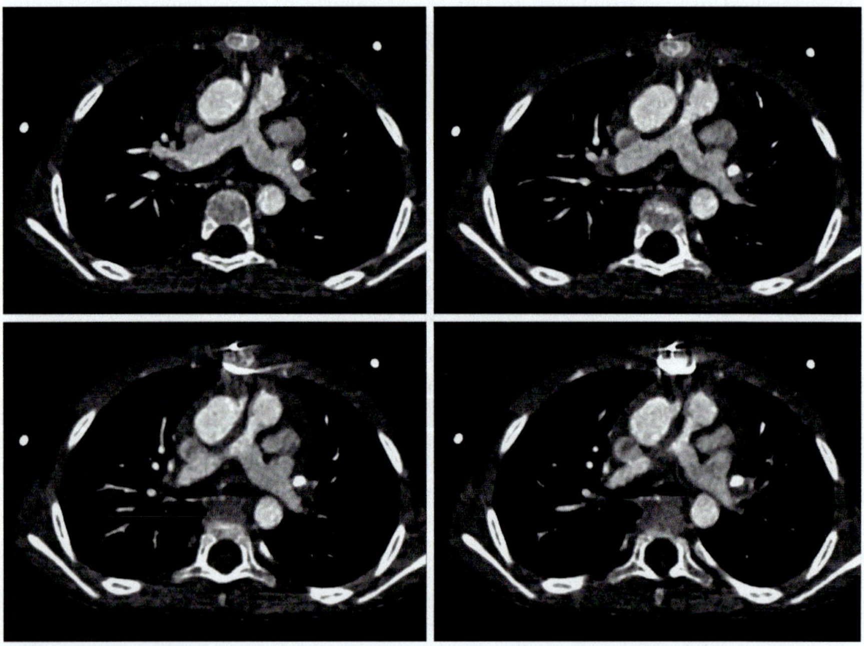

Fig. 33.2 Examples of axial CT images for a patient

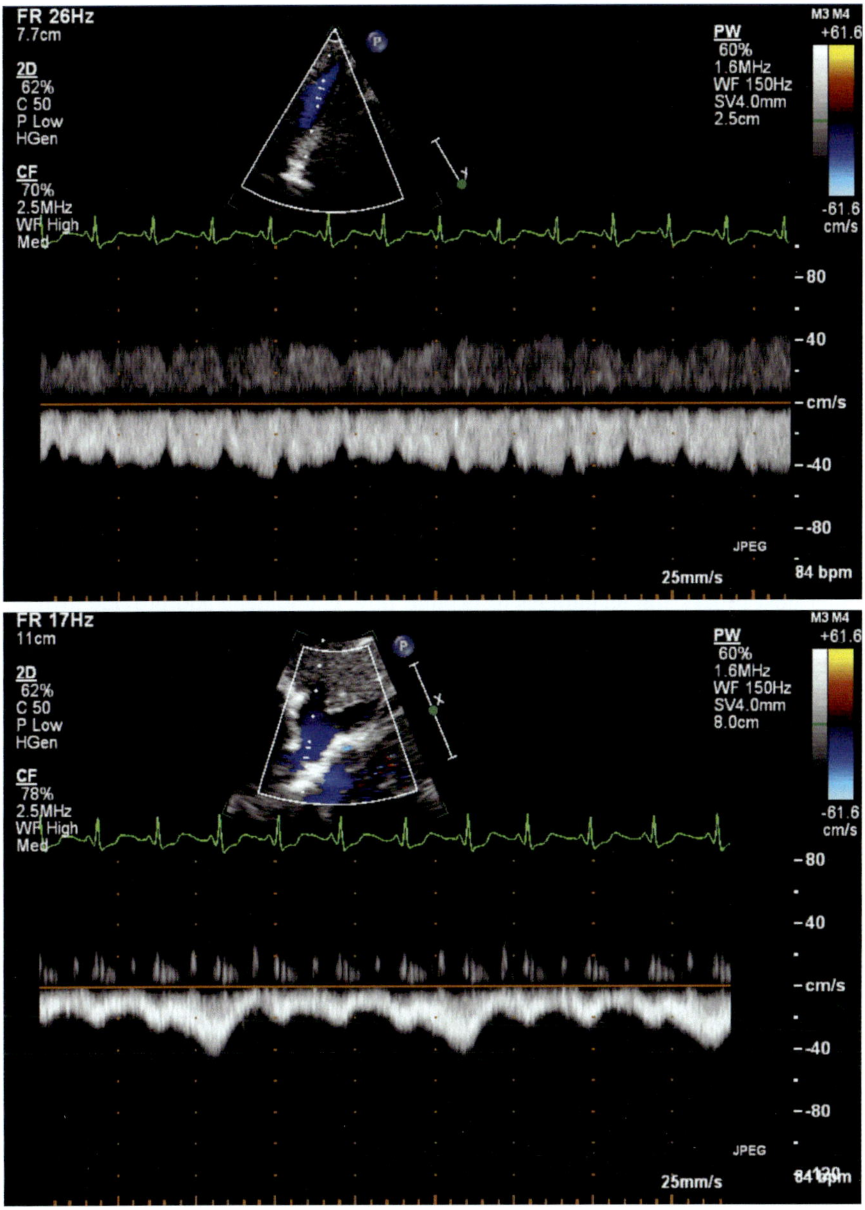

Fig. 33.3 Example of blood flow rate from echocardiography in superior vena cava (left) and inferior vena cava (right) for a patient with sinus rhythm

2003, 2008). Examples of commercial software include MIMICS (Materialise NV, Belgium) and GEOMAGIC (Geomagic Inc., NC, USA) for anatomical reconstruction and Medviso Segment (Medviso AB, Sweden) for flow segmentation.

Fig. 33.4 An example of a Glenn connection reconstructed from CT images

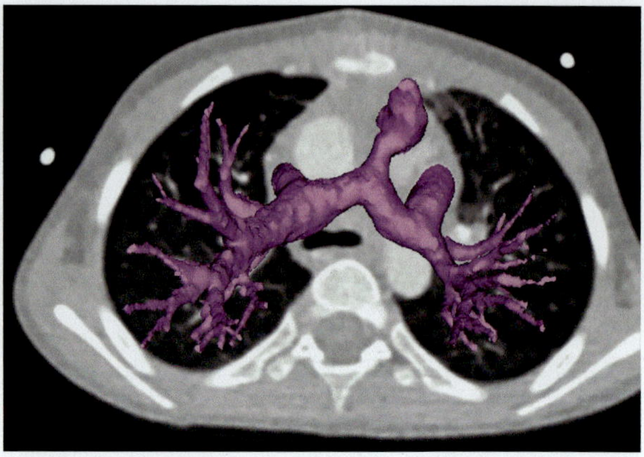

33.2 Computational Fluid Dynamics

CFD can be applied in a wide variety of disciplines, including, but not limited to, mathematics, fluid mechanics, and computer science. It utilizes visualization and other post-processing techniques to explore flow phenomena and provide insights for practical engineering/clinical purposes.

Fig. 33.5 illustrates a standard procedure used to set up a CFD simulation. Once the anatomy is defined, the next step involves mesh generation. In this step, the domain of interest, i.e., the anatomy, is "discretized" into a mesh. "Discretization" is a term used extensively in the field of CFD, and the mesh is composed of a cluster of elements, where each element is bounded by points (nodes). When creating the mesh, the domain of interest is actually a continuum that can be represented by an infinite number of elements. CFD solvers can then solve for flow quantities (e.g., velocities and pressures) at all these elements; however, using an infinite number is not a practical computational approach. Instead, one can prescribe a finite number of elements at which the CFD solver can obtain values of the flow quantities.

CFD solvers, in one form or another, are developed to obtain solutions of governing equations which represent physical laws of fluid motion. Three major governing equations for ICS are:

Continuity equation (conservation of mass):

$$\frac{\partial \rho}{\partial t} + \nabla \cdot (\rho \mathbf{u}) = 0 \tag{33.1}$$

in which ρ is density, and $\mathbf{u}$ is the velocity vector.

Navier–Stokes equation for incompressible viscous fluid (conservation of momentum):

$$\rho \frac{\partial \mathbf{u}}{\partial t} + \rho (\mathbf{u} \cdot \nabla) \mathbf{u} = -\nabla p + \mu \nabla^2 \mathbf{u} + \mathbf{f} \tag{33.2}$$

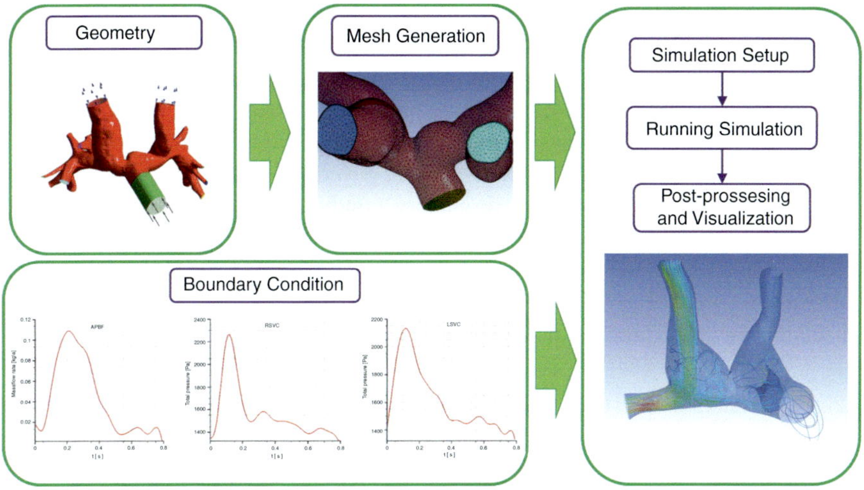

Fig. 33.5 A schematic of the standard procedure used for performing CFD simulations for single ventricle patients

in which p is pressure, μ is the viscosity, and $\mathbf{f}$ is the external force vector. This equation describes conservation of momentum per unit volume. On the left-hand side, the first and second terms represent the rate of increase of momentum and rate of momentum lost by convection, respectively. The first and second terms on the right-hand side stand for the changing rate of momentum because of pressure and shear stress, respectively.

Energy equation (conservation of energy) (Anderson et al. 1997):

$$\rho\left(\frac{\partial \varepsilon}{\partial t}+\mathbf{u}\cdot\nabla\varepsilon\right)=-\nabla\cdot\mathbf{q}+\Phi+S_{\mathrm{h}} \tag{33.3}$$

in which ε is the internal energy per unit volume, $\mathbf{q}$ is the heat transfer, Φ is the dissipation function, and S_{h} considers the external heat sources/sink. The physical meanings of the left-hand side terms are similar to that of conversation of momentum. On the right-hand side, the first term represents the rate of heat lost by conduction per unit volume. The heat transfer can be expressed as $\mathbf{q} = -k_{\mathrm{h}}\nabla T$ based on Fourier's law for heat transfer, in which k_{h} is the heat conductivity and T is the temperature. The second term corresponds to the changing rate of mechanical energy in the process of deformation of the fluid because of viscosity:

$$\Phi=\nabla\cdot\left(\overline{\overline{\tau_{ij}}}\cdot\mathbf{u}\right)-\left(\nabla\cdot\overline{\overline{\tau_{ij}}}\right)\cdot\mathbf{u} \tag{33.4}$$

in which $\overline{\overline{\tau_{ij}}}$ is the viscous stress tensor.

It is impossible to obtain exact solutions of these equations. Fortunately, many numerical methods can approximate their solutions by using a system of algebraic equations. Common methods for approximating solutions include the finite difference method (FDM), finite element method (FEM), and finite volume method (FVM). Each method employs a unique treatment of the mesh, which will be discussed in the next section. Nevertheless, these governing equations, by their nature, are partial differential equations. Boundary conditions are essential for solving these mathematical formulas.

By now, all the basic components for conducting a CFD simulation have been introduced. Once the simulation is finished, a myriad of flow quantities can be visualized through post-processing (Fig. 33.6).

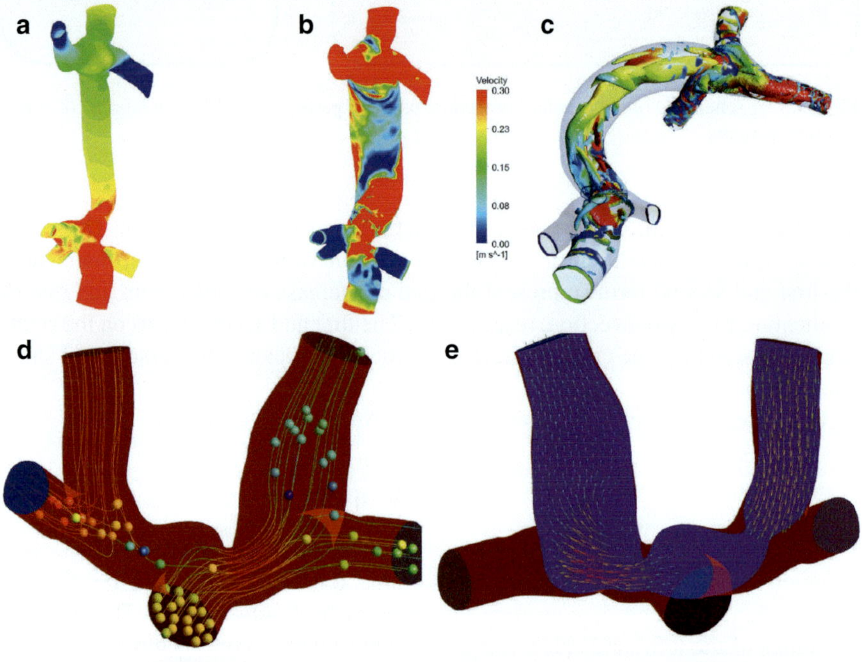

Fig. 33.6 Examples of post-processing for visualization of: (**a**) pressure contours, (**b**) wall shear stress, (**c**) vortex iso-surfaces, (**d**) streamlines, and (**e**) velocity vectors at a defined plane

References

Anderson DA, Tannehill JC, Pletcher RH. Computational fluid mechanics and heat transfer. 2nd ed. Oxfordshire: Taylor & Francis; 1997.

Frakes DH, Conrad CP, Healy TM, Monaco JW, Fogel M, Sharma S, Smith MJT, Yoganathan AP. Application of an adaptive control grid interpolation technique to morphological vascular reconstruction. IEEE Trans Biomed Eng. 2003;50(2):197–206. https://doi.org/10.1109/TBME.2002.807651.

Frakes DH, Dasi LP, Pekkan K, Kitajima HD, Sundareswaran K, Yoganathan AP, Smith MJT. A new method for registration-based medical image interpolation. IEEE Trans Med Imaging. 2008;27(3):370–7. https://doi.org/10.1109/TMI.2007.907324.

Wei ZA, Trusty PM, Tree M, Haggerty CM, Tang E, Fogel M, Yoganathan AP. Can time-averaged flow boundary conditions be used to meet the clinical timeline for Fontan surgical planning? J Biomech. 2017;50:172–9. https://doi.org/10.1016/j.jbiomech.2016.11.025.

Chapter 34
Overview of Image-Based Computational Simulation for Single Ventricle Hemodynamics

Zhenglun Alan Wei and Biao Si

34.1 Solver

Many CFD algorithms have been developed for engineering applications. Commercial solvers are widely used, and their engineering applications have been validated for decades. However, their applications regarding ICS are limited. One challenge of simulating single ventricle hemodynamics is properly representing the complexity of anatomic geometry and its corresponding moving parts. These moving parts, leading to a morphing mesh, are especially challenging using conventional CFD methods. Many state-of-the-art academic CFD algorithms have been introduced to address these challenges. Good examples are the immersed-boundary (IB) method, overset grid method, spectral method, and smoothed particle hydrodynamic method. However, these novel methods have their pros and cons. Therefore, proper validation against controlled experiments is always very necessary.

34.2 Geometry

Fluid dynamics are strongly dependent on the shape of the geometry. Therefore, a good geometrical representation of patient-specific anatomy is a key component of ICS, although idealized models were, historically, prevalent in many simplified numerical studies. A patient-specific anatomy gives full consideration to detailed

Z. A. Wei (✉)
Wallace H. Coulter Department of Biomedical Engineering, Georgia Institute of Technology and Emory University, Atlanta, GA, USA

B. Si
Fudan University, Shanghai, China

B. Qiao et al. (eds.), *Surgical Atlas of Functional Single Ventricle and Hypoplastic Left Heart Syndrome*, https://doi.org/10.1007/978-981-10-8435-5_34

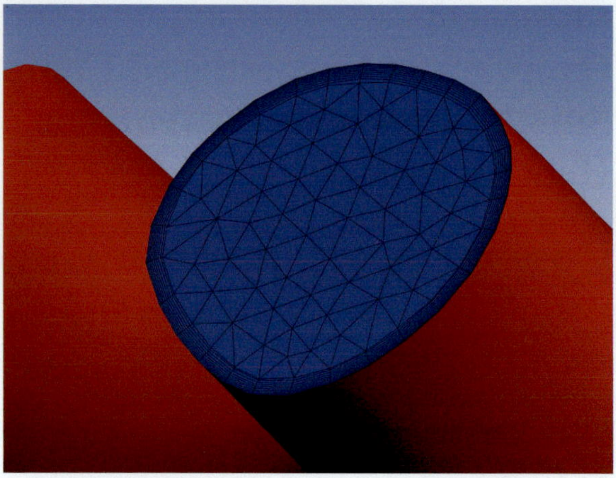

Fig. 34.1 An example of prism mesh near the vessel wall (green circle)

geometric characteristics of the vessel, including bifurcation, curvature, cavity, stenosis, etc. Accurate representation of the patient-specific anatomy plays an important role in the individualized diagnosis of disease and patient-specific surgical planning (Trusty et al. 2018).

34.3 Grid Generation

The computational grid is the discrete representation of the computational domain. A hexahedral mesh is often used for simple geometries, while an unstructured tetrahedral or polyhedral mesh is generally used with complex geometries. Polyhedral mesh is well-known for its fast convergence and low computational cost. However, a tetrahedral mesh is widely employed for its moving/dynamic grid method. Nevertheless, local grid refinement, e.g., prism mesh near a wall, is usually adopted to better resolve a large velocity gradient, as shown in Fig. 34.1.

Additionally, the quality of the grid directly affects the convergence and accuracy of the simulation. Therefore, a grid-independent study is the prerequisite to any computational study (Wei et al. 2017). In a grid-independent study, the grid is refined until the computed flow quantities of interest are not significantly affected by further grid refinement.

34.4 Boundary Conditions

A boundary condition (BC) is a series of known values at the boundary of the computational domain that drives the solution of the governing equations. The boundaries of the computational domain for single ventricle hemodynamics primarily include vessel walls and vessel ends.

34.4.1 BC for Vessel Walls

ICS often assumes rigid vessel walls. However, it is sometimes necessary to resolve the wall deformation to improve accuracy of the computed fluid dynamics in vessels or ventricles. Therefore, a fluid–structure interaction (FSI) model can be developed. To date, the most prevalent industrial FSI method is the Arbitrary Lagrangian-Eulerian (ALE) method. It, however, involves moving mesh and requires re-meshing that consume significant computational power. Therefore, the ALE method is not ideal for applications with large deformation. Alternatively, some state-of-the-art CFD algorithms, such as the IB method, have inherent advantages when dealing with largely deformed objects (Wei and Zheng 2017; Wei et al. 2014). It is worth noting that these state-of-the-art CFD algorithms are not universally superior for all FSI applications because of their own limitations (Wei et al. 2018).

34.4.2 BC for Vessel Ends

Clinical measurements are commonly imposed on the vessel ends as BCs. Though in vivo blood flow is pulsatile, time-averaged flow quantities are acceptable as BCs when the in vivo blood flow pulsatility is low. Simulations with time-averaged BCs benefit from fast computational time. Pulsatile flow BCs, on the other hand, are necessary to accurately simulate the fluid dynamics in the vessels, especially when resolving the effects of free-breathing and exercise (Wei et al. 2016). However, the drawback of using clinical measurements is that the simulated pressure field is only a relative pressure to a reference pressure unless invasive catheterization is employed. Absolute pressure is important for clinical diagnosis and FSI.

Alternatively, a cardiovascular lumped parameter network (cLPN) can be used to match both clinical flows and pressure measurements and provide physiological BCs to CFD solvers. In coupling with the CFD solver, the cLPN can model the responses of other organs and the entire body's circulation to the change in local hemodynamics simulated by the CFD solver. However, parameter estimation of cLPN and limited clinical inputs challenge its robustness.

34.5 Blood Model

In vivo blood is a non-Newtonian fluid, whereas it can be assumed to be Newtonian in regions of high shear rates. A non-Newtonian blood model includes, but is not limited to, the Carreau model and Casson model. More sophisticated methods can be used to include the effects of red blood cells and platelets, but with the added cost of increased computational resources.

References

Trusty PM, Slesnick TC, Wei ZA, Rossignac J, Kanter KR, Fogel MA, et al. Fontan Surgical Planning: Previous Accomplishments, Current Challenges, and Future Directions. J Cardiovasc Transl Res. 2018.

Wei ZA, Sonntag SJ, Toma M, Singh-Gryzbon S, Sun W. Computational fluid dynamics assessment associated with transcatheter heart valve prostheses: a position paper of the ISO Working Group. Cardiovasc Eng Technol. 2018.

Wei ZA, Tree M, Trusty PM, Wu W, Singh-Gryzbon S, Yoganathan A. The Advantages of Viscous Dissipation Rate over Simplified Power Loss as a Fontan Hemodynamic Metric. Ann Biomed Eng. 2017.

Wei Z, Whitehead KK, Khiabani RH, Tree M, Tang E, Paridon SM, et al. Respiratory effects on Fontan circulation during rest and exercise using real-time cardiac magnetic resonance imaging. Ann Thorac Surg. 2016;101(5):1818–25.

Wei ZA, Zheng ZC. Fluid-structure-interaction simulation on energy harvesting from vortical flows by a passive heaving foil. J Fluid Eng. 2017.

Wei ZA, Zheng ZC, Yang XF. Computation of flow through a three-dimensional periodic array of porous structures by a parallel immersed-boundary method. J Fluid Eng. 2014;136(4):040905.

Chapter 35
Clinical Applications of Image-Based Computational Simulation for Single Ventricle Hemodynamics

Biao Si and Zhenglun Alan Wei

35.1 ICS-Aided Clinical Study

ICS provides a very cost-effective means to understand patient-specific hemodynamics, thereby facilitating measurement of hemodynamic metrics for clinical studies which often involve a large population. With this approach, previous studies demonstrated that balanced perfusion to the left and right pulmonary arteries is of importance to the growth of the pulmonary arteries. It was found that the distribution of the hepatic factor to the left and right lungs, or hepatic fluid distribution, is linked to pulmonary arteriovenous malformations, a common long-term complication for Fontan patients. Moreover, the distribution of total pulmonary blood flow was associated with energy loss inside the Fontan and Glenn connection. Energy loss was hypothesized to be an important indicator of the exercise capacity of Fontan and Glenn patients. Reducing energy loss is a universal goal in single ventricle surgeries, especially for patients with hypoplastic left heart syndrome. The postoperative circulation of these patients often reveals low pressure and poor cardiac power, and is therefore susceptible to external disturbances, such as respiration and gravity.

B. Si
Fudan University, Shanghai, China

Z. A. Wei (✉)
Wallace H. Coulter Department of Biomedical Engineering, Georgia Institute of Technology and Emory University, Atlanta, GA, USA

B. Qiao et al. (eds.), *Surgical Atlas of Functional Single Ventricle and Hypoplastic Left Heart Syndrome*, https://doi.org/10.1007/978-981-10-8435-5_35

35.2 Surgery Optimization with ICS

Through knowledge gained by ICS-aided studies, ICS has also been adopted to assist clinicians in the optimization of existing surgical techniques and the exploration of novel surgery designs. The following section highlights several examples of this application.

Migliavacca et al. investigated different anastomosis types between the inferior vena cava and right pulmonary artery and concluded that an enlarged patch could lead to a more balanced blood flow distribution and lower energy loss. Ding et al. found that the flow collision between blood from the IVC and SVC determines the TCPC energy loss, and the anastomosis angle affects the hepatic fluid distribution (Ding et al. 2013). Tang et al. (2014, 2017) systemically studied the geometric characteristics of the TCPC and debated conclusions from Ding et al. by demonstrating that the minimum IVC diameter is the leading factor of TCPC energy loss and that the offset between the IVC and SVC primarily drives the hepatic fluid distribution.

Additionally, Lakshmi et al. conducted a comparative study between the extracardiac conduit and intra-atrial connection of the TCPC and revealed that a balanced total pulmonary blood flow benefits the cardiac output of the extracardiac TCPC (Dasi et al. 2011). Hsia et al. elaborated that a TCPC with a 20 mm diameter extracardiac conduit and left pulmonary artery anastomosis results in minimum energy loss (Hsia et al. 2004). Pekkan et al. found that a bidirectional Glenn connection has reduced energy loss compared to a Hemi-Fontan connection (Pekkan et al. 2009). Pekkan et al. studied the TCPC with bilateral SVCs and concluded that the optimal IVC anastomosis position for low energy loss is between the left and right vena cava (Zélicourt et al. 2006). Last but not least, Soerensen et al. employed ICS and prototyped the "OptiFlo," which is designed to achieve a good hepatic fluid distribution (Soerensen et al. 2007).

At the Institute of Cardiovascular Disease (ICD) of the General Hospital of Jinan Military Region, Jinan, China, the corresponding editor, Dr. Bin Qiao also utilized ICS to test some of his novel surgical ideas. For example, Dr. Qiao adopted an in-house design of an anastomosis that maintains the diameter of the vessel throughout its connection to the TCPC. An example of in-house design of an SVC anastomosis is illustrated in Fig. 35.1. This anastomosis is compared to a bulky anastomosis that has a remarkably larger size than the SVC diameter.

The anatomies in Fig. 35.1 were artificially made based on reconstructed CT images from a normal person without any congenital heart defects. Fig. 35.2 plots the streamlines obtained from ICS. It indicates a more chaotic flow pattern is formed with the bulky anastomosis.

This chaotic flow pattern in the bulky anastomosis results in more hotspots with high shear stress (Fig. 35.3) and oscillating shear index (Fig. 35.4), and two factors are unfavorable to normal physiology.

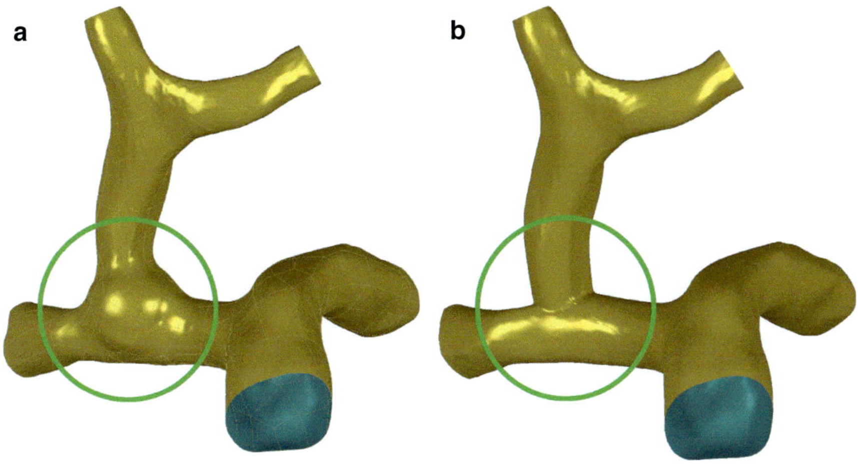

Fig. 35.1 An anatomic comparison between (**a**) a bulky anastomosis and (**b**) an in-house design of an anastomosis

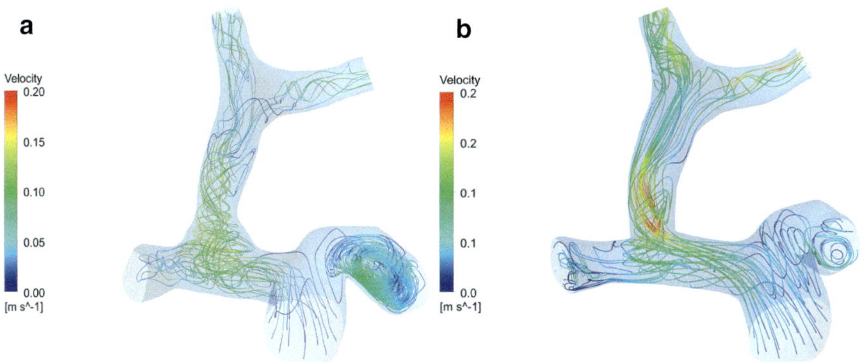

Fig. 35.2 Comparison of streamlines between (**a**) cavopulmonary anstomosis in which blood vessels are mismatched in diameter; (**b**) cavopulmonary anastomosis in which blood vessels are well matched in diameter

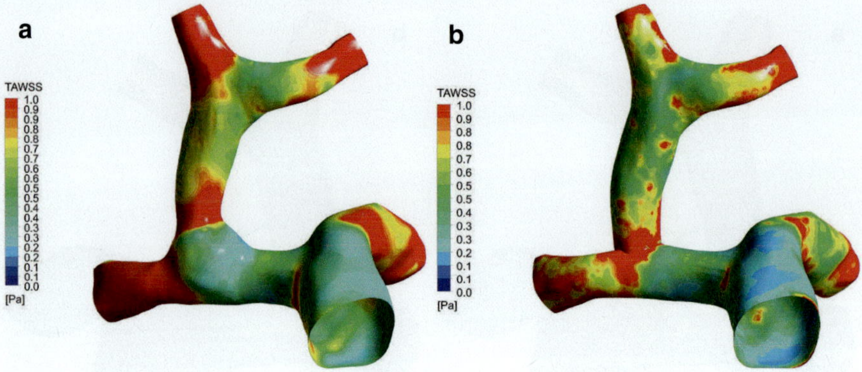

Fig. 35.3 Comparison of wall shear stress (TAWSS) contours between (**a**) cavopulmonary anastomosis in which blood vessels are mismatched in diameter; (**b**) cavopulmonary anastomosis in which blood vessels are well matched in diameter

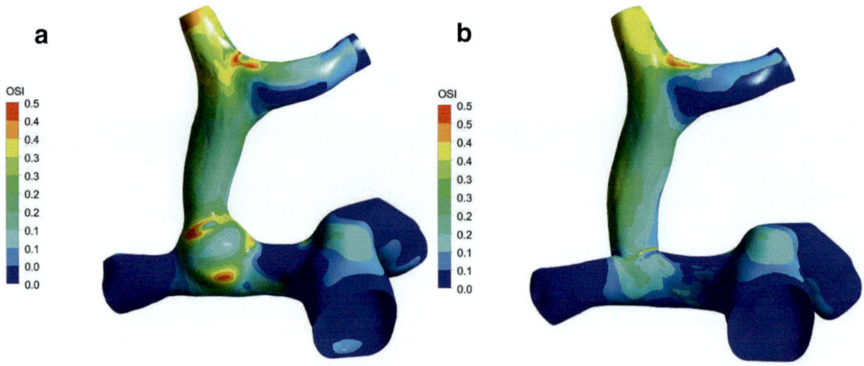

Fig. 35.4 Comparison of oscillating shear index (OSI) contours between (**a**) cavopulmonary anastomosis in which blood vessels are mismatched in diameter; (**b**) cavopulmonary anastomosis in which blood vessels are well matched in diameter

35.3 Virtual Surgical Planning

Virtual surgical planning by ICS fosters a close collaboration between engineers, clinicians, and surgeons, in order to come up with a defined clinical problem that is solvable based on ICS capacity and surgical planning time. The simulation setups must reflect the physiological state of the patients; however, necessary simplifications have to be made for the sake of meeting the clinical time frame. Clinicians and surgeons provide guidance for accurate reconstruction of the patient-specific anatomy and quantification of boundary conditions from medical images, as well as propose potential surgical strategies. Engineers then determine the appropriate computational approach for the clinical problem, evaluate the hemodynamic metrics of interest, and present the computed results to clinicians using visualization tools.

With the aid of virtual surgical planning, surgeons, clinicians, and patients can have improved understanding of the hemodynamic implications of the proposed surgical strategy prior to the surgery, thereby enhancing their confidence in the surgery and improving the success rate of the procedure. Nevertheless, it should be recognized that simulation results are imperfect because assumptions in model development as well as numerical errors are only approximations for in vivo flow features. There would therefore be gaps between any proposed strategies and their actual implementation. Fogel et al. (2013) qualitatively illustrated differences in the flow field between preoperative ICS predictions and postoperative MRI reconstruction while Haggerty et al. (2012) quantitatively demonstrated discrepancies in hepatic flow distribution. In addition to differences between pre- and postoperative flow conditions, they attributed this discrepancy to the inevitable variation between the proposed anatomy and the actual implementation performed by the surgeon. Restrepo et al. (2015) further investigated the effect of this anatomic variation and concluded that its effect is very patient-specific. Marsden (2013) proposed an uncertainty quantification approach to quantify numerous uncertainties involved in the virtual surgical planning. Mark et al. (Luffel et al. 2016) developed a novel platform, the Surgery Modeler (SURGEM), to facilitate the investigation of many uncertainties, thereby speeding up the virtual surgical planning process. Therefore, clinicians and surgeons should not treat ICS predicted hemodynamics as a gold-standard, but rather as a very important guideline. Their knowledge and experience should be used to examine and interpret the simulated results. The final clinical decision must be made by comprehensive understanding of ICS alongside a thorough consideration of the clinical condition of the patients.

35.3.1 A Sample Case at the Institute of Cardiovascular Disease

This section describes a sample case of a conducted ICS for surgical planning at the Institute of Cardiovascular Disease of the General Hospital of Jinan Military Region, Jinan, China. It compares the TCPC hemodynamics using two different sizes of Fontan pathways: 25 mm and 13 mm in diameter as shown in Fig. 35.5.

In Fig. 35.6, the simulation with a 25 mm pathway shows more recirculating flow compared to the simulation with its 13 mm counterpart. The 25 mm pathway therefore produces more clear vortex structures, as shown in Fig. 35.7.

Moreover, the case with the 25 mm pathway illustrates a large area of low shear stress (Fig. 35.8) and high oscillating shear index (Fig. 35.9), which are hypothesized to be correlated with the long-term development of anastomosis.

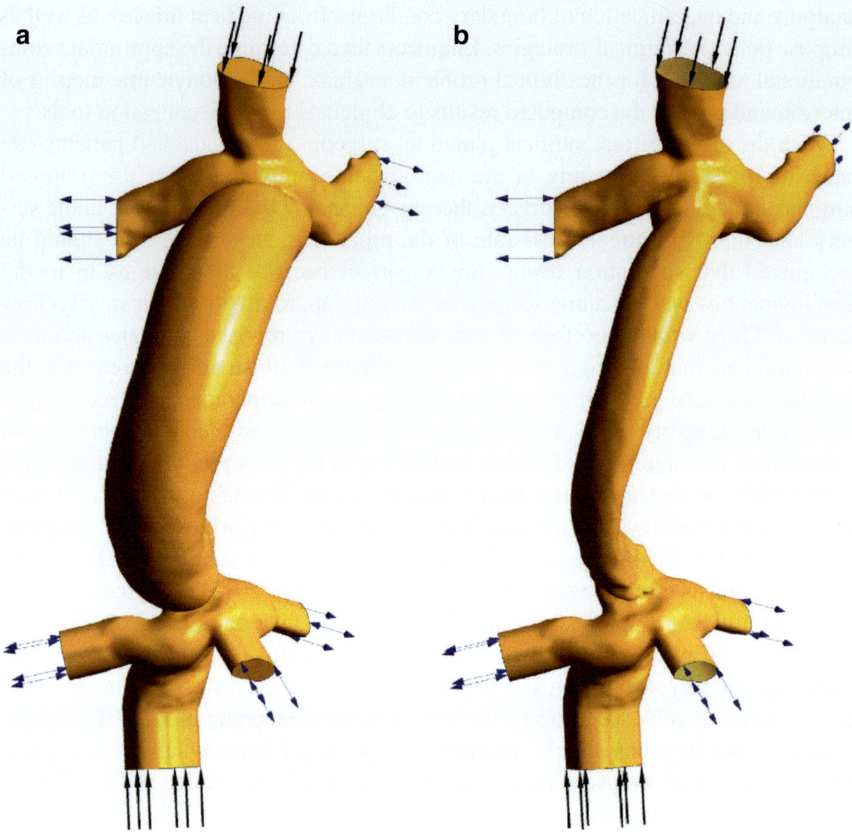

Fig. 35.5 Geometric comparison between (**a**) simulation with a larger extracardiac conduit (25 mm in diameter); (**b**) simulation with a smaller extracardiac conduit (13 mm in diameter)

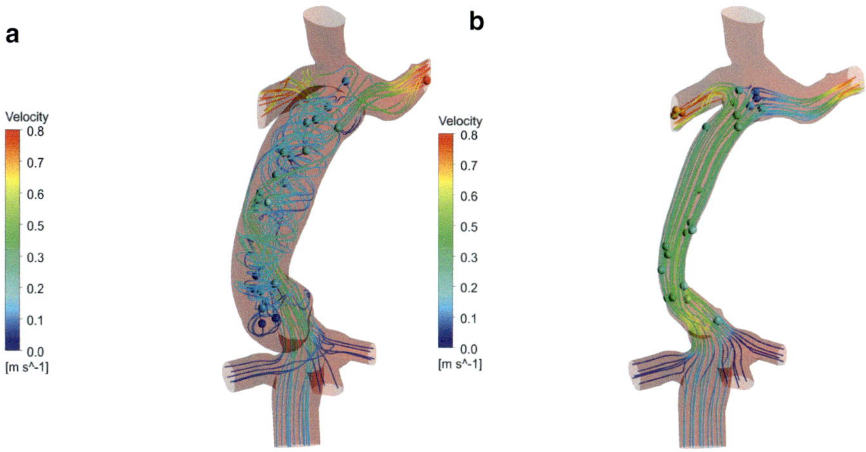

Fig. 35.6 Example comparison of streamlines between (**a**) a 25 mm diameter extracardiac conduit—recirculating flow; (**b**) a 13 mm diameter extracardiac conduit—linear flow is almost obtained

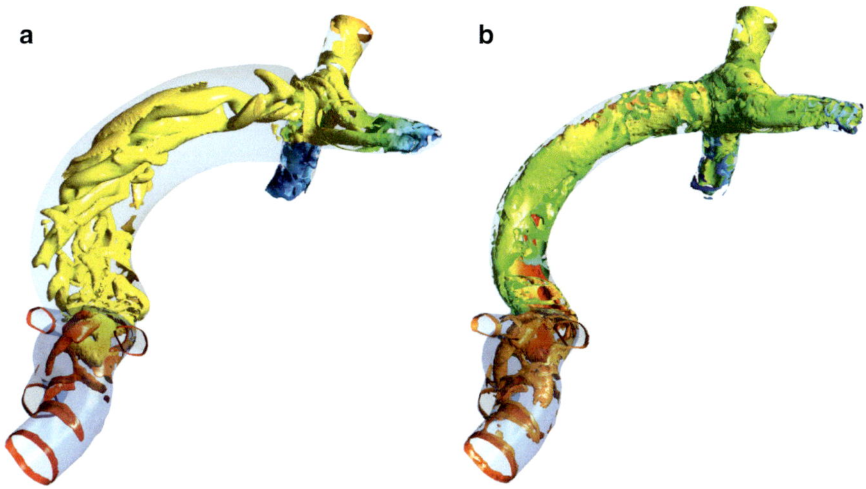

Fig. 35.7 Example comparison of vortex iso-surfaces between (**a**) 25 mm diameter extracardiac conduit; (**b**) 13 mm diameter extracardiac conduit

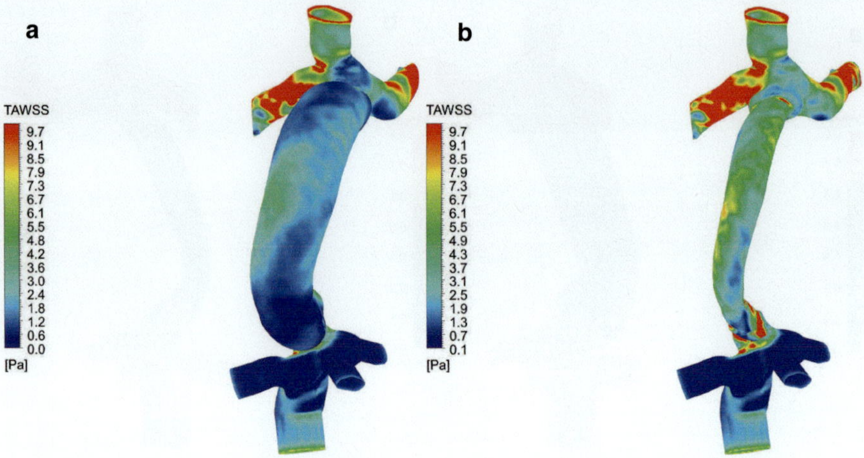

Fig. 35.8 Example comparison of distribution of wall shear stress (TAWSS) between (**a**) 25 mm diameter extracardiac conduit; (**b**) 13 mm diameter extracardiac conduit

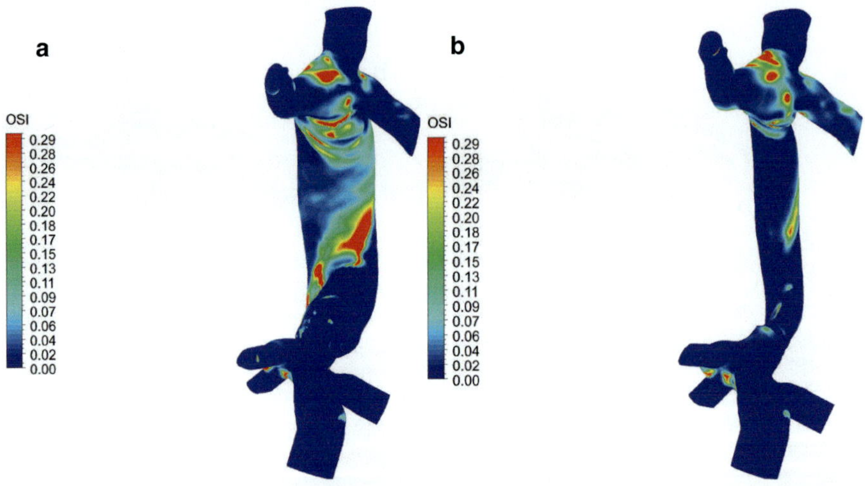

Fig. 35.9 Example comparison of the oscillating shear index (OSI) between (**a**) 25 mm diameter extracardiac conduit; (**b**) 13 mm diameter extracardiac conduit

References

Dasi LP, Whitehead K, Pekkan K, de Zelicourt D, Sundareswaran K, Kanter K, Fogel MA, Yoganathan AP. Pulmonary hepatic flow distribution in total cavopulmonary connections: Extracardiac versus intracardiac. J Thorac Cardiovasc Surg. 2011;141(1):207–14. https://doi.org/10.1016/j.jtcvs.2010.06.009.

Ding J, Liu Y, Wang F. Influence of bypass angles on extracardiac Fontan connections: a numerical study. Int J Numer Method Biomed Eng. 2013;29(3):351–62. https://doi.org/10.1002/cnm.2508.

Fogel MA, Khiabani RH, Yoganathan A. Imaging for preintervention planning: pre- and post-Fontan procedures. Circ Cardiovasc Imaging. 2013;6(6):1092–101. https://doi.org/10.1161/CIRCIMAGING.113.000335.

Haggerty CM, de Zelicourt DA, Restrepo M, Rossignac J, Spray TL, Kanter KR, Fogel MA, Yoganathan AP. Comparing pre- and post-operative Fontan hemodynamic simulations: implications for the reliability of surgical planning. Ann Biomed Eng. 2012;40(12):2639–51. https://doi.org/10.1007/s10439-012-0614-4.

Hsia TY, Migliavacca F, Pittaccio S, Radaelli A, Dubini G, Pennati G, de Leval M. Computational fluid dynamic study of flow optimization in realistic models of the total cavopulmonary connections. J Surg Res. 2004;116(2):305–13. https://doi.org/10.1016/j.jss.2003.08.004.

Luffel M, Sati M, Rossignac J, Yoganathan AP, Haggerty CM, Restrepo M, Slesnick TC, Kanter KR, del Nido P, Fogel MA. SURGEM: a solid modeling tool for planning and optimizing pediatric heart surgeries. Comput Aided Des. 2016;70:3–12. https://doi.org/10.1016/j.cad.2015.06.018.

Marsden AL. Simulation based planning of surgical interventions in pediatric cardiology. Phys Fluids (1994). 2013;25(10):101303. https://doi.org/10.1063/1.4825031.

Pekkan K, Dasi LP, de Zelicourt D, Sundareswaran KS, Fogel MA, Kanter KR, Yoganathan AP. Hemodynamic performance of stage-2 univentricular reconstruction: Glenn vs. hemi-Fontan templates. Ann Biomed Eng. 2009;37(1):50–63. https://doi.org/10.1007/s10439-008-9591-z.

Restrepo M, Luffel M, Sebring J, Kanter K, Del Nido P, Veneziani A, Rossignac J, Yoganathan A. Surgical planning of the total cavopulmonary connection: robustness analysis. Ann Biomed Eng. 2015;43(6):1321–34. https://doi.org/10.1007/s10439-014-1149-7.

Soerensen DD, Pekkan K, de Zelicourt D, Sharma S, Kanter K, Fogel M, Yoganathan AP. Introduction of a new optimized total cavopulmonary connection. Ann Thorac Surg. 2007;83(6):2182–90. https://doi.org/10.1016/j.athoracsur.2006.12.079.

Tang E, Restrepo M, Haggerty CM, Mirabella L, Bethel J, Whitehead KK, Fogel MA, Yoganathan AP. Geometric characterization of patient-specific total cavopulmonary connections and its relationship to hemodynamics. J Am Coll Cardiol Img. 2014;7(3):215–24. https://doi.org/10.1016/j.jcmg.2013.12.010.

Tang E, Wei ZA, Whitehead KK, Khiabani RH, Restrepo M, Mirabella L, et al. Effect of Fontan geometry on exercise haemodynamics and its potential implications. Heart. 2017;103(22):1806–12.

Zélicourt DAD, Pekkan K, Parks J, Kanter K, Fogel M, Yoganathan AP. Flow study of an extracardiac connection with persistent left superior vena cava. J Thorac Cardiovasc Surg. 2006;131(4):785–91. https://doi.org/10.1016/j.jtcvs.2005.11.031.

Chapter 36
Future Direction

Ajit P. Yoganathan and Guang Hong Ding

Both medical and economic concerns have stimulated the development of ICS for use in the cardiovascular system. It is a powerful tool for both biomedical research and clinical applications. ICS offers a promising means to cost-effectively examine and improve the performance of medical devices for the cardiovascular system, thereby reducing the cost of the product development process. Clinically, it is a noninvasive approach that can be used to augment other medical imaging and diagnostic techniques, thereby improving surgical outcomes and patient care. Moreover, ICS brings many new concepts to cardiovascular research, as well as applications such as virtual surgery, predictive medicine, and surgical planning. However, the complexity of the cardiovascular system poses unique challenges.

The primary challenge is that of validation. Variations in anatomy and flow conditions result in highly patient-specific flow conditions. Additionally, aging and growth are inevitable as many single ventricle patients are babies, adolescents, or young adults. ICS validation therefore becomes extremely challenging. Limitations may include the details of patient data available, especially follow-up surgical data, the number of patients, and the heterogeneity of clinical data acquired from different centers and patients. Therefore, a platform that shares unified patient data for research could benefit the ICS community.

The second challenge is computational speed. To accurately simulate physiological conditions, ICS requires several computational resources including memory,

A. P. Yoganathan (✉)
Wallace H. Coulter Department of Biomedical Engineering, Georgia Institute of Technology and Emory University, Atlanta, GA, USA
e-mail: ajit.yoganathan@bme.gatech.edu

G. H. Ding
Department of Mechanics and Engineering Science, Fudan University, Shanghai, China
e-mail: ghding@fudan.edu.cn

B. Qiao et al. (eds.), *Surgical Atlas of Functional Single Ventricle and Hypoplastic Left Heart Syndrome*, https://doi.org/10.1007/978-981-10-8435-5_36

computational power, and time. These delay the turnover time for ICS and prevent ICS from becoming a useful tool in the operating room. Fortunately, with growing computational power, parallel computing capacity, and the development of advanced algorithms, real-time ICS may come to be an indispensable clinical tool in the operating room.

Despite of resolving aforementioned challenges, many new techniques can be incorporated with ICS to further improve the clinical care and patient outcomes.

Virtual reality (VR) or virtual augmented reality (VAR) generates a virtual environment and gives the user direct access to interact with the environment. VR or VAR can be used to mimic the operating room and let surgeons practice operations virtually. ICS could then provide feedback to surgeons by evaluating their virtual surgery. Moreover, after surgical planning is performed using ICS, 3D printing technology could be used to print the proposed surgical connections or heart models to facilitate communication between clinicians and patients. With biocompatible materials, 3D printed models could also be directly used in patient-specific surgeries, thereby significantly reducing the surgery time, lowering the risk of the surgery, and improving the success rate of the surgery.

Abbreviations

ALE	Lagrangian-Eulerian
BC	Boundary condition
CFD	Computational fluid dynamics
cLPN	Cardiovascular lumped parameter network
CO	Cardiac output
CT	Computed tomography
DICOM	Digital imaging and communications in medicine
DORV	Double outlet right ventricle
FDM	Finite difference method
FEM	Finite element method
FSI	Fluid-structure interaction
FVM	Finite volume method
HLHS	Hypoplastic left heart syndrome
HR	Heart rate
IB	Immersed-boundary
ICD	Institute of Cardiovascular Disease
ICS	Image-based computational simulation
INV	Innominate vein
IVC	Inferior vena cava
LPA	Left pulmonary artery
LPM	Lumped parameter model
LSVC	Left superior vena cava
MPA	Main pulmonary artery
MRI	Magnetic resonance imaging
OSI	Oscillatory shear index
pcMR	Phase contrast MR
PDS	Polydioxanone suture
PLSVC	Persistent left superior vena cava

B. Qiao et al. (eds.), *Surgical Atlas of Functional Single Ventricle and Hypoplastic Left Heart Syndrome*, https://doi.org/10.1007/978-981-10-8435-5

PVR	Pulmonary vascular resistance
PVRI	pulmonary vascular resistance index
RPA	Right pulmonary artery
RSVC	Right superior vena cava
SV	Single ventricle
SVC	Superior vena cava
TA	Tricuspid atresia
TCPC	Total cavopulmonary connection
VAR	Virtual augmented reality
VR	Virtual reality
VR	Virtual reality
WSS	Wall shear stress

MIX
Papier aus verantwortungsvollen Quellen
Paper from responsible sources
FSC® C105338

If you have any concerns about our products,
you can contact us on
ProductSafety@springernature.com

In case Publisher is established outside the EU,
the EU authorized representative is:
Springer Nature Customer Service Center GmbH
Europaplatz 3, 69115 Heidelberg, Germany

Printed by Libri Plureos GmbH
in Hamburg, Germany